A Career Companion
to Becom

A Career Companion to Becoming a GP

Developing and shaping your career

Edited by

Patrick Hutt
BA, MBBS, DRSRH, MRCGP
Clinical Associate
UCL Research Department of Primary Care and Population Health
Salaried GP

and

Sophie Park
MBChB M.Med.Sci (dist) MRCGP (dist) DCH DFFP
Clinical Teaching Fellow in Primary Care
UCL Research Department of Primary Care and Population Health
Sessional GP

Foreword by

Roger Neighbour OBE
DSc, FRCGP, FRCP, FRACGP
Past President, RCGP

Radcliffe Publishing
London • New York

Radcliffe Publishing Ltd
33–41 Dallington Street
London
EC1V 0BB
United Kingdom

www.radcliffepublishing.com

Electronic catalogue and worldwide online ordering facility.

British Library Cataloguing in Publication Data

A catalogue record for this book is available from the British Library.

ISBN-13: 978 184619 553 2

Typeset by Phoenix Photosetting, Chatham, Kent
Printed and bound by Cadmus Communications, USA

Contents

Foreword

As I mouse-click a 'New Document' into being in order to write this Foreword, the thought hits me: What a cheek! What an irony! Here am I – drawing my NHS pension, my 30 years of clinical practice now well behind me – presuming to front a book telling you, one, if not two, generations younger than myself, why you might like to consider a career in general practice. What do *I* know about it anymore? *I* don't have to contend with Modernising Medical Careers and the European Working Time Directive; with the new MRCGP exam and revalidation; with practice-based commissioning and the Quality and Outcomes Framework; with the spectre of medical unemployment; with the morale-sapping corruption of professional judgement by pragmatic political imperatives. The real authors of this book, who are even now effectively sculpting their own careers amidst such turbulence, are far better qualified than I to tell it like it is.

So, I ask myself, why was I invited to make this contribution, and why did I agree?

I'm immodest enough to hope that I might be perceived as speaking up for something worth hanging on to in general practice, during times of change. And what is that 'something'? I have always believed that medicine is as much an interpersonal discipline as a scientific one, and that, among all the medical specialties, it is general practice that best allows the flourishing of both the doctor-as-scientist and the doctor-as-compassionate-human-being. General practice is at least as much about what PG Wodehouse's Jeeves called 'the psychology of the individual' as it is about the anatomy of the carpal tunnel or the latest revision to the guidelines for the treatment of hypertension. And why did I agree to write this Foreword? Because my own career as a GP has been satisfying beyond all my undergraduate imaginings, and I wish for nothing more earnestly than that some of you might share the deep-going joy of general practice, which is, knowing you have made a real difference in the lives of some of the individuals who have put their trust in you.

The one disappointing thing about a career in general practice is sometimes having to explain why it is so rewarding. Sadly, the stereotype still persists that general practice is for the 'also-rans'. This misconception has its origins in history, as does the reality that general practice nowadays is where some of the best doctors are to be found.

In 1958, the Royal Commission on Doctors' and Dentists' Pay heard evidence from the then President of the Royal College of Physicians, Lord Moran. The following exchange took place:

> *The Chairman*: 'It has been put to us by a good many people that the two branches of the profession, general practitioners and consultants, are not senior or junior to one another, but they are level. Do you agree with that?'
> *Lord Moran:* 'I say emphatically "No!" Could anything be more absurd? I was Dean at St Mary's Hospital Medical School for 25 years, and all the people of outstanding merit, with few exceptions, aimed to get on the staff. It was a ladder off which they fell. How can you say that the people who fall off the ladder are the same as those who do not?'

Lord Moran subsequently attempted to retract, explaining that he had merely sought to improve the financial lot of junior hospital doctors, who spent long years in training on low salaries. But his talk of a 'ladder' had touched a nerve. For like most insults, it contained a degree of truth.

The National Health Service had been established in 1948. In its early years, there was an undeniable status gradient between, at one extreme, the god-like teaching hospital consultant with his retinue of sycophantic and ambitious underlings and, at the other, the single-handed provincial family doctor, well-meaning and popular, but often clinically inept. Nonetheless, Lord Moran's analysis – that all doctors aspired to be consultants, and it was only those who couldn't make the grade who ended up in general practice – was an over-simplification. Would-be consultants were motivated by more than the drive for clinical supremacy; greed and vanity were often in the mix as well. And, it was not just low-achievers who became GPs; many chose general practice because it was a family tradition, or for its comfortable way of life, or out of a genuine belief that medicine was a humanitarian cradle-to-grave commitment.

So, the effect of Lord Moran's remarks on general practitioners – or at least on those who were proud of the under-recognised achievements of family medicine and who appreciated its potential as an essential counterpoise to the hospital services – was to galvanise them into action. The College (later Royal College) of General Practitioners (RCGP), which had been founded in 1952 despite fierce opposition from the Royal College of Physicians, realised that only a sustained drive to establish the defining hallmarks of good general practice, and to guarantee appropriate training in its core skills for all new GPs, would salvage the reputation and future of the discipline. On both counts, it was spectacularly successful. Responding to Moran's assertion, Dr John Horder, one of my own mentors who later became President of the RCGP, wrote in its Journal:

> Specialists expect to remain under part-time training until they are from 33 to 40 years old. Is it surprising that some of them have feelings of superiority – and some of us feelings of inferiority – when our own training is so much shorter? Unless this differential is altered what right have we to expect much change in the other differential?

And so, as it turned out, we have good reason to be grateful to the noble lord for his rudeness. It has had three enormously valuable results over the subsequent decades.

Firstly, it stung the ever-growing number of GPs who took their medical skills seriously into action. They and their academic body, the RCGP, recommitted themselves to proving an old truth – that clinical generalism and clinical competence were not mutually exclusive. General practice could be the nursery of medical excellence, not its graveyard.

Secondly, it prompted GPs to clarify what were the defining characteristics of good general practice. The GP might indeed be the jack of all medical trades; but he (it was usually 'he' at that time) was also the master of one – the open-ended and unconditional medical care of the uniquely individual patient.

Thirdly, it spurred GP educationists within the RCGP to pioneer the UK's system of vocational training for general practice. They devised its curriculum; they built up the educational expertise and infrastructure required to deliver GP training on a national scale; they lobbied successfully for the necessary political support and funding. The result has been that, in terms of educational quality, postgraduate training for general practice overtook that for the hospital-based specialties more than 30 years ago. And it has maintained that advantage. The UK's system of vocational training in the specialty of general practice is now incontestably the finest in the world.

These three – insistence on high clinical standards, the recognition of clinical generalism as a specialty in its own right, and a commitment to excellence in training – are the legacy which those of you who are contemplating a career in general practice stand to inherit. Let's look a little more closely at each, to satisfy ourselves that this is more than empty rhetoric.

Hospitals increasingly restrict their activities to the highly specialised, high-tech resource-heavy end of the healthcare spectrum. The corollary of this is that patients who need less intensive care increasingly receive that care within the purlieu of general practice. Most routine care of patients with hypertension, coronary artery disease, dyslipidaemias, mental health problems, diabetes, obstructive airways disease, and other chronic conditions is now undertaken in primary care. Most practices can swiftly access the whole gamut of investigations and diagnostic procedures, and offer additional services such as minor surgery, contraception or counselling. As long as this increase in responsibility can be matched by assurances as to quality – and it can – there are clear advantages to all parties. Patients benefit from convenience and continuity of care. Hospitals are freed to concentrate their resources where they are most effective. GPs have the opportunities to reinforce and extend their clinical skills. And the NHS delivers better value for the taxpayer.

There have been both sticks and carrots in the process of raising clinical standards in general practice. On the 'stick' front, all new entrants to general practice must now meet the exacting requirements of the MRCGP assessment, and will (as all doctors will) subsequently have to submit themselves and their clinical outcomes to the scrutiny of revalidation. 'Carrot'-wise, practising to high clinical standards has become its own reward. A critical mass of GPs now take professional pride in their ability to deliver uncompromisingly competent clinical care. The days when the GP dealt with only the most minor of illnesses, and referred anything the least bit complicated to the hospital, are gone. Increasing numbers of GPs, for example, are seeing some value in becoming 'GPwSI's – GPs with a special interest – working in hospital, in tandem with consultant colleagues from a wide range of specialties. This hybrid role allows both specialist and generalist to respect and learn from each other's skills. While a few pockets of poor general practice admittedly remain, they will not long survive the professional climate change of continuous improvement that is now well under way.

Moving on to consider the assertion that 'general practice is a clinical specialty in its own right'; you might perhaps think this is something of a contradiction in terms. Perhaps your medical education to date has led you to think that general practice is no more than the sum of all the little bits of low-level specialist knowledge needed to get through a working day, with a dash of business management and administration thrown in. This would be a misunderstanding. While, of course, the GP's clinical knowledge is only a small subset of the collective experience of all the specialist disciplines, there is a fundamental difference between how generalists and specialists each set about their medicine. The difference is one of perspective.

Faced with a clinical problem, the specialist's usual response is to zoom in on its detail and examine it, as it were, through a close-up lens. The specialist will explore the minutiae of a disease, even if that means (and it often does) filtering out many of the individual patient's unique features. To the specialist in diabetes, focusing on abnormal function in the islet cells of a patient's pancreas, the fact that the owner of that pancreas might be depressed, or unemployed, or the father of a child with learning difficulties, is of passing interest only. The generalist, on the other hand, faced with the same patient, will also 'pull back' and view the bigger picture as if through a wide-angle lens. To the generalist, context and interconnectedness are as important as detail. In the generalist's way of thinking, illness is more than just a biological malfunction. It is inseparable from the patient's psychological, social, family, environmental, financial, even spiritual circumstances. The GP's 'big picture' care of that diabetic patient will, of course, include regularly monitoring blood sugar control, adjusting medication and checking for complications. But it will also extend to addressing the depression that might undermine his compliance with treatment, and referring him to an occupational health department to discuss alternatives to his previous job as a lorry driver. It is likely, too, that the same GP will know the patient's wife and child, and be able to anticipate the ramifications of his diabetes on the relationships within an already stressed family.

The 'open access' nature of general practice means that GPs may see illness at a very early stage in its natural history, often before typical diagnostic features have had time to emerge. Managing this clinical uncertainty calls for a sensible balance between over- and under-investigation, and for a nicely-judged feel for the appropriate use of time to make things clear. One further point of difference between the clinical spectrum seen by specialists and GPs is that patients, particularly older ones, often suffer from more than one disease at once. Managing this co-morbidity calls for sensitivity and compromise; the GP will understand that the best treatment for a patient with angina, hyperlipidaemia, irritable bowel disease and osteoarthritis is not necessarily the sum of the ideal treatments for each condition.

One of the most important conceptual differences between the generalist and specialist ways of practising medicine lies in how each sees the role of the relationship between doctor and patient. Conventional 'specialist' wisdom is that any psychological transactions between them are at best a distraction from, and at worst a threat to, the effectiveness of the medical agenda. The generalist, on the other hand, knows that such a detached position is neither possible nor, indeed, desirable. On the contrary; the doctor's understanding of the psychosocial roles that doctor and patient adopt, and of the nuances of communication between them, can be a valuable source of diagnostic insight and therapeutic leverage. If you come into general practice, you will find that much attention is paid during your training to acquiring 'consulting skills', so that you can effectively manage the communication process within the consultation, and are not scared to allow 'yourself-as-a-person' into the consulting room as well as 'yourself-as-a-doctor'.

I don't wish to give the impression that clinical diversity, 'wide angle' thinking and psychological astuteness are the unique preserve of general practice. Many good specialists try to remember that the patient is a complex and multidimensional individual. It's just that a true generalist can never forget it, and wouldn't want to.

You'll learn more in later chapters in this book about what is involved in specialty training for general practice. You will also receive a well-informed sense of the world of contemporary general practice which might await you. It is undeniably a more complex, more diverse, more hard-nosed and more uncertain world than that which I entered in 1974; but it is no less rich in challenge and reward. That is also true of hospital medicine. The relentless increase in medical knowledge, achievement and expectation affects primary and secondary care alike. But technological advances make it harder, yet no less important (I believe), to preserve the compensatory effect of the generalist's 'big picture' perspective. Person-specific pharmacology; genome-based therapies; surgical nanotechnology – we are awash with medical advances offering the beguiling but, ultimately, false hope of near-perpetual health. Combine this mirage with the cacophony of official voices claiming to know what is best for us, and, back in the villages and housing estates where real people live, the need for medical professionals with common sense and a personal touch, whom people can trust and talk to, is obvious.

So – have you got what it takes to practise the 'medicine plus' which is today's general practice? This book, written and edited by colleagues many of whom have far more street cred than I, will help you decide. If you have, I wish you luck, fulfilment, and the gratification that comes from being a catalyst for good in the lives of your fellow human beings. If you have a role teaching and mentoring the next generation of GPs, you will find this book a persuasive ally. But if you decide that hospital medicine is your preferred option – well, that's fine. There would be no shame, if you find the ladder to general practice too steep, in settling for becoming a brain surgeon.

Whatever you decide, medicine is the best job in the world. Have a great career.

Roger Neighbour
Bedmond
May 2011

About the editors

Patrick Hutt qualified as GP in 2008 and has written various articles about general practice. He is author of *Confronting an Ill Society*, a biography of David Widgery; a radical East End GP. He is Deputy Editor of *InnovAiT*, the RCGP journal for GP trainees. He is a Clinical Associate at UCL Research Department of Primary Care and Population Health and works as a salaried GP in Hackney.

Sophie Park is a practising GP in Hertfordshire. She teaches with UCL Medical School, the London Deanery and Institute of Education (IOE) at both undergraduate and postgraduate level in a variety of subjects relating to general practice and medical education. She co-ordinates community based placements for undergraduates in Dermatology, Child and Women's Health, teaches the iBSc in Primary Care Consultation module at UCL, and is a tutor on the Education and Technology in Clinical Practice MA, at the IOE. She contributed to the PasTest *'Practical guide to Medical Ethics and Law'* and is chapter author of 'The Industrialisation of Medical Education?' in *'Policy, Discourse and Rhetoric: how New Labour challenged social justice and democracy'* (Lall, M., Sense Publishing). Sophie's research for her EdD at the IOE includes exploring how undergraduate medical students develop their professional identity using narrative analysis.

List of contributors

Chapters 2 and 6

Mareeni Raymond MBBS BA (Hons) MRCGP DRCOG DFFP is currently an Academic GP ST4 at UCL Medical School. Mareeni did most of her Foundation Year training at the Whittington Hospital, North London, and her GP specialist training at the Homerton, East London, before returning to UCL for her ST4 year. She has an interest in teaching and writing, and has written a book for patients, *Coping with Life After Stroke*.

Joe Rosenthal BSc MSc MBBCh FRCGP DRCOG DFFP is Senior Lecturer in General Practice and Sub-Dean for Community Based Teaching at UCL Medical School, Programme Director for the Royal Free GP Specialty Training Programme and a part-time GP Principal in North London. He was lead editor of the book *Registrar's Companion for General Practice*.

Chapter 3

Judith Harvey MA DPhil BM BCh DRCOG started out as a research scientist, then taught in a comprehensive school in Liverpool and ran a volunteer programme in Papua New Guinea, before studying medicine. She has been a GP partner, a salaried GP and a locum. She has chaired a Local Medical Committee, sat on the General Practitioner's Committee of the British Medical Association, and was a member of the Council of the National Association of Sessional GPs. She writes regularly on sessional GP matters.

Chapter 4

Jennifer Chodera currently works as a locum. She started making films in 2005 when taking a year out from medicine to attend art school. She continues to pursue her interests in art and psychoanalysis in her spare time.

Chapter 5

Dominic Roberts was trained and currently works in Hackney, East London. He is a GP Principal in a large inner city practice and also works as a GPwSI in

ENT seeing patients from the local area, alongside a consultant, Mr Eynon-Lewis. Dominic helped to set up his local GPwSI clinic and has embraced the challenge and clinical variety this has brought. He enjoys bridging the gap between primary and secondary care and sharing his knowledge through teaching the primary care team and specialist general practice training programme. He is also involved as presenter for the BMJ Masterclass course on ENT in primary care.

Chapter 7

Andrew Dicker MBBS MA MSc has worked as a GP in central London for the past 20 years. He is a Programme Director for the London Deanery, a GP trainer and an accredited Balint Group Leader.

Chapter 9

Luisa Pettigrew MBChB MRCGP DFFP DRCOG DCH is a sessional GP in London. She developed a passion for International Health becoming involved with Medsin as a student in Edinburgh. She has undertaken a diploma in International Health and an MSc in Health Policy, as well as working in Latin America with NGOs and as an expedition medic. She helped form the RCGP Junior International Committee and currently coordinates the 'Hippokrates' international exchange programme through WONCA's Vasco da Gama Movement.

Iona Heath CBE MRCP PRCGP worked as an inner city GP at the Caversham Group Practice in London from 1975 to 2010. She chaired the RCGP International Committee until 2009 when she was elected as President of the Royal College of General Practitioners. She is a member at large of the WONCA world executive and has written extensively about general practice.

Foreword writer

Roger Neighbour MA MB Bchir DRCOG FRCP PRCGP has been a GP, trainer and Course Organiser in Hertfordshire; Convenor of the MRCGP Panel of Examiners; and President of the RCGP from 2003 to 2006. He is the author of *The Inner Consultation*, *The Inner Apprentice* and *I'm Too Hot Now*. Now retired from clinical practice, he continues to write, teach and lecture in the UK and worldwide on consulting skills and medical education.

Acknowledgements

Creating this book has been an affirming process for us both as GPs and academics. It has stimulated many conversations and questions, which we hope have enriched the text, as well as our own practice with patients and students. We are indebted to all those authors who have contributed so generously to this book, sharing their varied insights and experience. All the authors of chapters, career profiles and reflective pieces are General Practitioners reflecting on their own practical experience. In addition, we would like to thank our families, friends and each other for offering their endless support, encouragement and patience throughout this endeavour. We are grateful to our colleagues whose ongoing teaching, conversations and role-modelling have, of course, influenced our current vision of our professional world and practice, and would like to thank, in particular, Dr Joe Rosenthal at the UCL Research Department of Primary Care and Population Health.

CHAPTER 1

Introduction to general practice

Patrick Hutt

'The essence of general practice is an unconditional and open-ended commitment to one's patients'

McWhinney, 2003

This book is aimed at helping you decide about a career path in general practice and the various options within it. It is hoped that whatever path you choose, it will prove to be stimulating and rewarding. Careers are rarely well-formed from the outset and develop over time to meld with personal circumstances and emerging professional interests. In this chapter, you will be introduced to some definitions of general practice, taken on a historical whistle-stop tour involving a famous detective and provided with an overview of how to approach using this career book to best suit your individual needs.

What is General Practice?

This is an important question. There are constant attempts to articulate what general practice is and what general practitioners do. A lot of understanding about general practice draws heavily upon traditional views and perceptions about the family doctor. In the UK, relatively recent debates about general practice have often referred to a book entitled *A Fortunate Man: The Story of a Country Doctor*, written in 1967 by John Berger and the photographer Jean Mohr. For many people this book inspired them to become General Practitioners (Hutt, 2005).

A Fortunate Man is a poetic account of a doctor working in a rural community. General practice is shown to be hard work but as a job provides an intimacy with people's lives. This proximity to people's lives is sometimes difficult to appreciate from the outside looking in. At one point in the book, the analogy is drawn between the General Practitioner and the Master Mariner – who steer communities and ships through difficult seas.

Dr Sassell, the subject of the book, draws upon memories of doctors from his own childhood:

> 'a man who was all knowing but looked haggard. Once a doctor came in the middle of the night and I could see that he slept too – his pyjama trousers were poking out from the bottom of this trousers. But above all I remembered he was in command and composed – whereas everybody else was fussing and agitated.'
>
> Berger, 1967, p. 53

Some might argue that this is a rather romantic notion of a GP (though perhaps all images from childhood are). Certainly, the concept of doctors as 'all knowing' has been shaken due to the increasing complexity of disease management and the plethora of publicly accessible information resources. The doctor's pedestal has also decreased in height due to a number of high profile cases of problem doctors. GPs today are rarely responsible for their patients twenty-four hours a day, seven days a week. Rather than committing to one area for thirty years, GPs today often have portfolio careers – combining various roles with the more traditional one of patient care. It is nevertheless acknowledged that general practice is a stressful job (RCGP, 2005).

The Royal College of General Practitioners (RCGPs) defines general practice in the following way:

> General practitioners (GPs) are best defined by the unique nature of the doctor-patient relationship. GPs are personal doctors, primarily responsible for the provision of comprehensive and continuing medical care to patients irrespective of age, sex and illness. In negotiating management plans with patients they take account of physical, psychological, social, and cultural factors, using the knowledge and trust engendered by a familiarity with past care. They also recognise a professional responsibility to their community. GPs exercise their professional role by promoting health, preventing disease and providing cure, care or palliation. This is done either directly, or through the services of others according to health needs and the resources available within the community they serve.

During a career in general practice, it is common to experience challenges to this definition, both positive and negative. GPs may find that on some mornings there is little room for negotiation with patients. There may be times when GPs think of patients as friends or enemies, often within the space of one afternoon. General practice can be the best and worst job in the world. Arguably, it is during the course of a medical career that individuals reach their own understanding about what it means to be a General Practitioner. Like any good medical textbook, it is regularly updated.

One of the most daunting things about choosing a career path in general practice is the uncertainty. How do you know what will be required from the job in ten years? Will there even be jobs available in the place you wish to live? Will the things that drew you towards the profession still be part of the job requirement? We hope now to convince you that change is constant, a dynamic that, once embraced, can lead to opportunity and fulfilment.

Many moons ago…

If ever you find yourself becoming tired in a medical library, your eyelids heavy as you revise a complex clinically relevant topic – perhaps the Krebs Cycle, Vitamin D metabolism, or the local fertility referral pathway – try the following exercise. Stand up and proceed to the dustiest section of the library, where the journals that date from almost one hundred years ago, slightly worn around the edges, live. Pick up a volume, choose a page at random, and spend five minutes reading. You are unlikely to find the answer to the MRCGP exam questions, but there will be a refreshing sense of perspective.

The role of the General Practitioner emerged as an amalgamation of the skills of the apothecaries, who prescribed medicines and had to belong to a register (in contrast to quacks) from the early 19th century onwards; and the barber surgeons who were very 'hands on', sometimes with a saw. Today, it is often proudly quoted that half of all medical students go into general practice but similar figures were being quoted almost 100 years ago (BMJ, 1925). In short, the profession of General Practice had been shaped and evolved over many years.

Now for the detective story: At the end of the 19th Century, following completion of his medical training at the Royal London Hospital, Sir Arthur Conan Doyle, who was to later author Sherlock Holmes, was looking for a job as a General Practitioner. Jobs in London were hard to come by so he moved to Plymouth joining a partnership with another doctor that was unpleasant enough to make him leave promptly (Coren, 1995). In need of work, Conan Doyle moved to Portsmouth and set up a practice on his own which involved renting a house, furnishing a consulting room in the front and living meekly in the back. It took time to establish a reputation as a doctor in a new town. Business was slow. When there was an accident outside his house, he was the first on the scene and anonymously called the local paper to inform them of his success in a bid to generate custom. In his first year in practice he earned £154, then £250 and in his third year this rose to £300 (Booth, 1997).

Why mention this story? GPs at this time, like most of the medical profession, were generally men. General practice was competitive: unable to establish a successful practice in an oversaturated London market, Conan Doyle needed to move to earn a living. Even so, the living that he did make was relatively meagre and he needed support from other family members. Doctors had to build up their reputation to attract customers, which was especially difficult if starting up a practice from scratch. Doctors have not always been guaranteed a good living. An illustration from 1875 shows a group of doctors wearing top hats, walking through the streets begging, such was the explosion in the number of doctors training at this time (Digby, 1999). The National Insurance Act of 1911, and subsequently the advent of the National Health Service of 1946, went someway to ensuring that General Practitioners were assured of a regular income, although this was subject to fluctuations.

Today, there is similar turbulence surrounding job certainty in general practice, though not on such a scale. For example, at the time of writing, openings for GP partnerships are hard to come by, but in the 1990s were extremely hard to fill. This should not be of grave concern to someone considering a career in general practice. There is usually great demand for enthusiastic and committed GPs throughout the UK, not forgetting the rest of the world.

As Roger Neighbour highlights in the Foreword, general practice has had to battle against the perception that it is inferior to Hospital Medicine and Surgery, in order to be considered a specialty in its own right. This has led to some quite flamboyant defences of general practice. William McCartney, a GP in the United States, wrote in 1938 about General Practitioners as one might describe a Knight:

> 'Such courageous souls, battling more or less single-handed with pain, torment and suffering, fighting the grim reaper, that spares not the head of the large family, the sole wage earner, the mother with her manifold duties and responsibilities, or the only beloved child, need no apologist.'
>
> McCartney, 1938

It is hoped that collaborative care and integrated training has broken down some of this tribalism. However, recent experience of medical students and junior doctors suggests that some historical shadows persist. In extremis, such views are likely to be highly prejudiced. On my own travels I have listened to a hospital consultant proclaim that 'GPs are the greatest barrier to good medical care in the UK', whilst half a mile away a GP will state in a practice meeting, 'We'd be better off without any hospital doctors interfering with our patient care.' One should try to understand where these opinions come from, but equally, remember that good patient care requires both groups to work together.

Using this book

As editors, we are aware there is a need to outline in broad terms, the different career paths available, and to provide a space for you to consider what these might mean to you. We have resisted the temptation to produce a 'cook-book', informing you how to get from A–B. Inevitably there is an element of this, but we have encouraged our authors to write more widely, using their own experience as GPs, to illustrate their writing. Equally, readers must feel free to dip into those sections most relevant to their particular needs. Alongside our more traditional chapters, we have included accounts of career profiles, to illustrate the variety of career paths taken. We hope that these convey something of the breadth of possibilities available. Where there might be a danger that these profiles are too narrow in their scope, we have included short reflective pieces asking GPs to ponder explicitly upon their career path, or a moment within their career, that they feel might be salient. For example, 'What does it feel like to retire?' or 'What is it like completing GP training while bringing up a young family?' Where such reflections refer to patient interactions, their identity has been disguised. Most of our authors are from across the UK, but not all. Look out for a career profile intended to convey the international parallels with UK general practice.

We hope that this book will act as a springboard, to spark the imagination and encourage you to pursue the answers to your own questions. Applying to medical school, many are asked 'Why do you want to study medicine?' A decision to enter general practice should not be without similar consideration. Permutations on the same question continue to have relevance at different stages of a career. 'Why did you apply to become a General Practitioner four years ago?', 'What would you like to change about your GP career?' and 'Why support others to become a General Practitioner?' are useful reflective exercises. The importance of pausing to check your direction every so often cannot be underestimated. One definition of 'career' means to 'run at full speed' (OED, 1989). This is fine if you are confident that you are heading in the right direction.

The chapter about GP Training hopes to convey a sense of the modern hurdles that must be jumped to gain entry into the increasingly competitive training programmes. Written by a final-year current trainee, and an experienced GP educator, this should provide a broad understanding of the process rather than a 'how to' guide on completing the application form. The chapter also gives you a flavour of the structure of GP training as well as the numerous parts of the assessment process that must be completed before being 'qualified.' It is hoped that the experience of training to become a General Practitioner has evolved significantly beyond that described by David Morell who entered general practice in 1957, 'My vocational training lasted three days, because one of the partners was in desperate need of a holiday and left a week after my arrival.' (Morrell, 1998).

Of course, there is an argument that GPs are never truly qualified, as they are perpetually learning. There has long been a feeling that undergraduate training, and even vocational training, does not fully equip you for the challenges during lifelong practice. Unlike today, in the late 19th Century and early 20th Century, there were few courses that GPs could attend in order to maintain their knowledge; some doctors even booked locums so that they could spend a couple of weeks attached to a hospital (Digby, 1999, p. 61). Due to the breadth of knowledge required to be a GP, it has been recommended by the Tooke report that GP training should increase from three years to five, in line with other specialty training (Tooke, 2008). However, this and revalidation plans develop – the process by which GPs will demonstrate that they are competent to continue to practice during their career – doctors will be perpetually required to demonstrate they are reflective learners. Andrew Dicker's chapter on professional development provides a thought-provoking insight into how GPs might consider this aspect of their career development. Establishing good habits now will serve you well throughout your career, even if the exact shape the future will take remains unknown.

Permutations of provision

For most of the 20th Century, the typical working arrangement was for GPs to have control of their premises, either working alone or in partnership. This has changed dramatically, with more and more salaried posts available. Judith Harvey, a GP with experience of both arrangements, explores the historical context behind this shift in working patterns, which has led to something of a professional divide between salaried doctors and partnerships, and turns a constructively critical eye to both; challenging, for example, the assumption that taking a partnership at your training practice is necessarily the dream job.

One of the career pathways often overlooked is working as a locum. Jennifer Chodera, someone who has fashioned a successful locum career combined with making documentary films, stresses the potential wealth of knowledge and experience that a period spent working as a locum can provide. Follow her advice and you begin to see that working as a locum need not mean second-rate practice and poor working conditions. Her chapter also covers the increasingly segregated out-of-hours care, and considers how the type of medicine practised here varies from day-to-day practice.

General practice in the latter half of the 20th Century prided itself on the fact that 'generalism' was a 'specialism.' Today many people are excited about a career in general practice thanks to the potential to develop a special interest, which has led to new acronyms such as GPwSIs (GPs with a Specialist Interest). Traditionally within group practices, it has been natural for GPs to develop individual expertise and interest in specific health conditions, strengthening the resources of the team. With more and more services being moved from hospitals into the community, Dominic Roberts (a GPwSI in ENT) and Sophie Park explore the boundaries of generalism and specialism, and the potential to train and start up new services in what is a relatively new territory. Currently, many of the opportunities to provide specialist services are about how you network effectively with the organisational framework within your local area.

Teaching, research and travel

The Hippocratic Oath places great emphasis on the role of the medical teacher and encourages practitioners of medicine to share their knowledge.

> 'I hold him who has taught me this art as equal to my parents and to live my life in partnership with him, and if he is in need of money to give him a share of mine, and to regard his offspring as equal to my brothers in male lineage and to teach them this art – if they desire to learn it – without fee and covenant; to give a share of precepts and oral instruction and all the other learning to my sons and to the sons of him who has instructed me and to pupils who have signed to covenant and have taken an oath according to the medical law, but to no one else.'
>
> Ludwig, 1943

Thankfully, the medical profession today is far more open and diverse than the sentiments that might be understood from the above abstract. For those who think they are interested in teaching, or would simply like to try it out, then general practice provides a wealth of opportunities to get involved, from having medical students visit for a few days during the year, or to becoming a GP trainer.

Many trainees find that the close relationship with their trainer during their third specialist training (ST3 or 'registrar') year can provide a very broad and influential education, in what continues to be a modern day apprenticeship. As David Widgery, a GP and political activist, wrote of his GP trainer, 'He and I would have long philosophical arguments about art, politics and history in the Venus Steak House during our lunch hours. He would tell me about the imperfectability of human nature and reminisce about Bethnal Green in the days of the Krays.' (Widgery, 1991)

Sophie Park, a GP involved in clinical practice, teaching, and in the midst of her research for an education doctorate, discusses the teaching paths available to General Practitioners. She points out some of the training courses available, and suggests practical solutions to the common problems GPs face when having students visit their practice.

In the past, there has been a dearth of research opportunities available in general practice – with most research in the community being conducted by enthusiastic individuals with sporadic links to academic departments. The need to maintain an evidence base that reflects the nature of the problems facing general practice is critical and Mareeni Raymond – who has experience as an academic trainee – outlines the different career paths available, and how you might begin to explore the academic opportunities open to you.

There can be no doubt that a career in general practice spent solely on the shores of the UK is probably slightly colder than one spent in the rest of the world. One of the most rewarding and exciting ways to invigorate your career is to become involved in international work. We are privileged to have two authors, Luisa Pettigrew and Iona Heath, who work on the RCGP International Committee, writing about the ways in which GPs can begin to have an international outlook, whether it is by taking part in an exchange during your GP training, or using some of the highly valuable and transferable skills as a GP to work for a Non-Governmental Organisation (NGO). It can be incredibly refreshing to hear how other countries revere UK general practice and the NHS, or to see how some of the perceived impossibilities of your role are universal.

Deciding on a career in General Practice

Choosing a career path is not simple. For many people, it can be an agonising decision simply to apply to medical school. The assumption is often that once this decision has been made, the trajectory is clearly mapped. During my first year at medical school I was quite taken aback by students who appeared to be confidently marching towards haematology or neurosurgery. Not possessing such certainty, and struggling to recite the branches of the brachial plexus, I wondered whether medicine was for me. I asked my supervisor, Dr Ashley Moffet, what the best thing would be to do. Wisely, she replied 'It's probably time you thought about what **you** want, not what others are doing. The great thing about the medical profession is that there is something in it for everyone.'

If this is true for the medical profession more widely, it is especially true for those in general practice. This book attempts to highlight the diverse nature of the many roles available. One of the best pieces of advice for those considering a career in general practice is to ask other people about their jobs and career pathways. Such people can provide a wealth of information and anecdote. Nevertheless, remember this note of caution: when listening to people talk about their careers, it is often a story written backwards, told after they have arrived, settled and made themselves comfortable. For example, 'It was natural that I should have become a fulltime GP partner while I completed a PhD. I raised a family while completing my training and I still run a successful consultancy company. In my spare time, I run marathons to raise money for the animal sanctuary I set up.'

It is hoped that the pages of this book will provide you with some space to reflect on what is involved when undertaking a career in general practice. Perhaps one of the most liberating notions is that some of the best-laid plans fall by the wayside. Ask around. How many people ended up in their roles thanks to a faint breeze nudging them in a given direction? How many successes resulted from failure? Some of the most successful practices were built up from nothing, and some of the happiest doctors spent time not being doctors. Despite the element that fate plays in career paths, it is prudent to make plans. The career pathways are today arguably narrower in the wake of Modernising Medical Careers and the new RCGP curriculum. If you are aware of the options available now, it is possible to explore paths earlier, or accrue the experience required in order to facilitate a particular decision or direction.

If, after weighing up all the options, you still find yourself struggling to make a decision, perhaps consider the *Book of the Samurai*, which states that all decisions should be made within seven breaths (Tsunetomo, 2002).

Whether or not a career in general practice is associated with the adjuncts of teaching, research or international collaboration, general practice still provides a significant opportunity to make a difference to the lives of people on a very human level. It is hoped that this book will emphasise that there is no single 'career in general practice'. There are as many paths as there are doctors.

References

Berger J. *A Fortunate Man: Story of a Country Doctor* London: Penguin; 1967.
BMJ. The profession of medicine. *BMJ*. 1925; **2:** 405–410.
Booth M. *Doctor, the Detective and Arthur Conan Doyle: A Biography*. London: Hodder & Stoughton; 1997.
Coren M. *Conan Doyle*. London: Bloomsbury; 1995.

Digby A. Doctors Differ, A scene in Dr Richardson's City of Health, Chorus of Medical Practitioners, 'We have no work to do!' *The Evolution of British General Practice 1850–1948*. Oxford: Clarendon Press; 1999.

Hutt P. GPs fortunate or unfortunate? *BMJ Careers*. **331** (75177517); 2005.

Ludwig E. *The Hippocratic Oath and Johns Translation and Interpretation*. Baltimore: John Hopkins Press; 1943.

McCartney W. *Fifty Years and Country Doctor*. New York: Dutton and Company Inc.; 1938.

McWhinney I. The essence of general practice. In: Lakhani M, editor. *A Celebration of General Practice*. Oxford: Radcliffe Medical Press; 2003.

Morrell D. Introduction and Overview. In: Loudon I, Horder, K, Webster C, editors. *General Practice under the National Health Service 1948–1997*. Oxford: Clarendon Press; 1998.

OED. *Oxford English Dictionary*, 2nd edn. Oxford: Oxford University Press; 1989.

RCGP. *Stress and General Practice – Information Sheet 25*. [Online]. Available at: www.rcgp.org.uk/pdf/ISS_INFO_22_FEB05.pdf (accessed 25 July 2010).

Tooke J. *Aspiring to Excellence, Final Report of the Independent Inquiry into Modernising Medical Careers*; 2008. [Online]. Available at: www.mmcinquiry.org.uk/draft.htm (accessed 25 July 2010).

Tsunetomo Y. *Hagakure: The Book of the Samurai* (W. S. Wilson, trans.). Europe: Kodansha; 2002.

Widgery D. *Some Lives! A GP's East End*. London: Sinclair and Stevenson; 1991.

Career profile:

Chris Kenyon

When did you qualify?
1972 Royal Free Hospital MB BS
1984 MRCGP

What is your job?
I am a GP Principal at Grove House Surgery, Shepton Mallet, a GP specialist in Substance Misuse, a GP trainer and I volunteer with Festival Medical Services for the Glastonbury Festival.

Why and how did you choose General Practice?
I tried hospital jobs for five years: A&E, 18 months of paediatrics and community paediatrics, obstetrics and gynaecology for one year, then I spent four years working in Asia. I thought about a career in tropical medicine when I returned but felt England was where my home, family and cultural roots lay. General practice was the only area that could match the breadth of experience I wanted.

Where have you worked?
During four years in Asia, I travelled from London by motorcycle. In Tehran, I found work as a medical SHO (Notre Dame Di Fatima Hospital), India with Tibetan refugees, Thailand with Cambodian Refugees in paediatrics through an American aid organisation, then back to India and the Tibetans. I did medical work but also advised on water supplies, sanitation, solar heating projects and a cheap healthy diet. I found that I gained credibility within communities through my skills as a doctor.

I considered India as a place to live but decided England was home. I worked for one year as a GP registrar with Dr Hodgson in Finsbury Park (John Scott Health Centre), which was the beginning of my understanding of what general practice was about. GP locums prior to this had been like outpatient clinics. My GP registrar colleagues at the Homerton Hospital (Hackney Scheme) were an inspiring group.

I will always be grateful to my trainer Lewis Hodgson for encouraging me to attend a Balint Group at the Tavistock Clinic. That was a weekly commitment for many years with Dr Manny Lewis, a psychoanalyst, leading the group of GPs. It has ensured every consultation is at least interesting.

My first GP Principal position was at The Well Street Surgery in Hackney. I was very fortunate, one partner became the first Professor of General Practice at Barts, two partners had MRCPsych, and four partners out of six had been involved in Balint Groups. Paul Julian remains a mentor and inspiration. We were a teaching practice with a family atmosphere for medical students and trainees. Wednesday 8.30am clinical meetings were inspiring.

A six-month sabbatical in 1994, stimulated thoughts of the future and family discussions led to a move out of London to Somerset via six months' travelling with my two children, aged six and eight. My registrar at the time became a partner.

Where do you work?
It took me longer than expected to find a practice, but by 1997 my wife and I were appointed as a job share at Grove House Surgery, Shepton Mallet.

We work together in a five-partner practice: I do six sessions; my wife five. I am a trainer and do one session a week as a clinical specialist in substance misuse.

Each year, the Glastonbury festival appears in our practice area. Through the charity Festival Medical Services we provide care to a city of 180 000 people who suddenly appear in Pilton; with the associated births and deaths, trench foot and sunburn it is perhaps the safest place in the country for a 'bad trip'. Equally, we get to listen to the legends. In 2008, Leonard Cohen brought my daughter to tears and took me back to teenage years with *Suzanne.*

What is the most rewarding aspect of your job?
I believe everyone has a story to tell. Balint has refined that for me, and I treat medical problems on the way. I feel privileged to be close to people when they are dealing with major life events like death, birth, and cancer. The practice is like a family, working together to provide the best healthcare possible for our local community, supporting each other, learning together exchanging ideas, and having fun. Sometimes we 'cure people' but most often we listen.

GP training and education provide challenges and much pleasure. Working with Substance Misuse, I find I am working with often-marginalised people at high risk of death. Achieving stability can be a real achievement, sometimes they even move on. Hepatitis C and HIV remain significant challenges.

Retirement is in sight and we are planning a new surgery; to hand over to a new partner with a new surgery built would be a dream.

What is the most challenging or frustrating thing about your job?
The growing number of patient contacts is pushing the increasing number of administration tasks into the early morning, evening or weekend. Access, as the government's prime indicator of quality, conflicts with continuity of care

which I believe to be more important. The future of general practice remains uncertain; is it to be the partnership model, where all doctors have a stake in the practice, or one where larger private companies employ salaried doctors and nurses?

If you could change one thing about your career what would it be?

I wish I had attempted to make contact with general practice during my medical student days or hospital jobs in the 1970s, as a mentor for me at that time could have been significant.

What do you wish you knew then that you know now?

I wish I had understood what general practice was about much earlier in my career: every patient has his or her story.

Reflective piece: 'Why general practice? Why me?'

Ronald MacVicar

Why medicine? Why general practice? Why me? These are all important questions, especially for me; the fourth of four siblings, all of whom studied medicine and all of whom became general practitioners. Counter-intuitively, I think it was harder than it seems to settle on the same career as my siblings; I struggled constantly against the notion that I was simply following suit or suffered from some lack of imagination.

So, where did my desire to be a GP come from? It was later in my career that I realised it probably came from my father. He was a Presbyterian minister on the Isle of Skye and approached the pastoral element of his role with real commitment. He visited and comforted the sick, he assiduously visited parishioners who were in hospital some three hours drive away in Inverness. He was a major part of most families' crises and their celebrations. He was a non-medical role model for a model general practitioner.

So, I trained for general practice, returned to the Highlands and joined a busy small practice in Inverness. A passion for teaching and learning drew me towards training and eventually into the postgraduate educational system. I was appointed as Director of Postgraduate General Practice Education (DPGPE) for the North of Scotland Deanery in 2008. This role has dragged me away from general practice for all but one day per week. This is a day that is precious, that grounds me and that gives me some credibility in my other role; a credibility that is needed more internally than externally I suspect.

Being the DPGPE for a vast area like the North of Scotland has its challenges as well as its joys. Recruitment to training in the north is challenging despite the fact that feedback on our programmes is highly positive. Many newly qualified doctors seem to want to stay in the west end of some city or other and commute to work which, for a boy from Skye, is hard to understand. In contrast, opportunities exist for our trainees to experience work and life in some of the most beautiful parts of the world with unrivalled access to outdoor and sporting pursuits, cultural and historical tradition and high measures of quality of life. And in my role I get to visit them or the places that they work.

I think of a storm brewing in the darkening sky viewed from the surgery window of our most northerly training practice in Shetland. I think of a spectacular winter sunrise over the Western Isles when

INTRODUCTION TO GENERAL PRACTICE **15**

coming in to land for a day visit to our team there. I think of the spectacular scenery and history evident in a drive between Oban and Lochgilphead hospitals. I think of the Stone Age settlements and Viking runic carvings in Orkney and feel a sense of connection and continuity; perhaps part of the connection and continuity that passed from my father to me.

Once people come to live and work in the Highlands and Islands, they usually stay. I did, and I cannot imagine living anywhere else. But sshhh… don't spread it around too much, there isn't room for everyone!

CHAPTER 2

General practice specialty training

Mareeni Raymond and Joe Rosenthal

What is specialty training?

In order to practise as an NHS General Practitioner, you will need to complete a minimum of a three-year period on a recognised GP Specialty Training Programme (GPSTP) and gain the nMRCGP qualification. This must be preceded by completion of a medical degree and a two-year Foundation Programme or its equivalent. Candidates who successfully complete the nMRCGP and obtain a licence to practise, are eligible for inclusion on the General Medical Council's GP Register and for membership of the Royal College of General Practitioners (RCGP). Most GP training programmes now include 18 months in hospital-based training posts combined with 18 months based in general practice. Some four-year training programmes are available and there are proposals that all programmes should move to four or even five years in the future (Tooke, 2008).

This chapter will briefly outline the history of specialty GP training, the process of applying for training, the structure of the training programme and assessment procedures along the way. At the end of the chapter, you can read one trainee's account of their experience during their specialist training. Do not be daunted by what might seem a long and complex process. If you are sure general practice is the career for you, then the rest should be plain sailing.

History of specialty training

Specialty Training used to be called Vocational Training; a term initially used in the 1960s when the RCGP first introduced the concept of specific postgraduate training to become a GP. In 1978, it became a requirement for a doctor to complete one year of supervised training in general practice before practising independently as a GP. Prior to this, any doctor could work as a GP partner, assistant or locum. In 1983, the training period was extended to three years of which one year had to be spent in a training general practice and the other two years in a variety of approved hospital posts. Accreditation followed satisfactory completion of the required experience and there was no compulsory qualifying exam. The MRCGP examination did exist at that time but as an optional test, which could be taken by GPs at any point in their career in order to demonstrate excellence and gain membership of the RCGP.

In 1997, a process of compulsory Summative Assessment (SA) was introduced to provide objective testing of GP registrars' skills, ensuring that those completing training had achieved a minimum level of competence. The SA process included four elements: a Multiple Choice Questionnaire (MCQ), an assessment of consultation skills using video or simulated surgery, a written submission of practical work (e.g. a clinical audit or project) and a structured trainer's report.

In 2007, SA was replaced by nMRCGP as the new single assessment system for GP training. The process focuses on competencies and consists of three elements: an Applied Knowledge Test (AKT), a Clinical Skills Assessment (CSA), and a Workplace-Based Assessment (WPBA). Evidence of achievement of the required competencies is collected in an on-line portfolio (e-portfolio) which is reviewed regularly by the trainee and their supervisor, and yearly by the Deanery Annual Review of Competence Progression panels (ARCP). This ensures that a trainee is meeting the required standards before continuing to the next stage of training and eventually gaining a Certificate of Completion of Training (CCT). This will be explained in more detail later in this chapter.

Applying for General Practice training

Since February 2006, there has been a centralised national process for applying to GP training in the UK, which is managed by the GP National Recruitment Office on behalf of all the UK deaneries. To be eligible to apply, the candidate must have a primary medical qualification, be fully registered with the UK GMC at the time of application or have passed both parts of the Professional and Linguistic Assessments Board (PLAB) exam and be eligible for full UK GMC registration at the time of applying. The candidate must have achieved Foundation competencies during their foundation years one and two, and should be able to demonstrate proficiency in English language. They have to be eligible to work legally in the UK.

Training posts are advertised each December or January for the following August intake. Application can only be submitted on-line and programmes are available at ST1 to ST3 level. The National Recruitment Office for General Practice Training website (www.gprecruitment.org.uk) lists which posts are available in which deaneries around the country. Applicants are advised to read the individual deanery profile pages and access individual deanery websites for more information about programmes available in each area. Applicants can rank up to four deaneries in order of preference. A small number of Academic Clinical Fellowship (ACF) Programmes are also available in some deaneries. Applications are not accepted for a planned deferred start date unless they are registered for a higher degree.

Selection process for GP training

There is a competitive and complex selection process for specialty training, arguably more rigorous than other specialty application processes. It involves:

Stage 1: On-line application form.

Stage 2: Machine Marked Test (MMT). Once your application is accepted you will be asked to attend an initial assessment, which forms the short-listing process. This assessment is conducted under examination conditions and you will be asked to agree to a set of rules before you can proceed. This first assessment is conducted on one day in deaneries across the UK and you will be able to attend at the closest available centre to where you are currently living. The assessment consists of two papers to be completed under invigilated conditions. The papers are designed to assess the essential competencies in the National Person Specification (*see* www.gprecruitment.org. uk for further details) and are based around clinical scenarios.

The first paper (two hours) covers Professional Dilemmas and requires candidates to rank possible solutions to problems in order of appropriateness. The second paper (90 minutes) is on Clinical Problem Solving and includes questions based on clinical scenarios which require you to exercise judgment and problem-solving skills to determine appropriate diagnosis and management of patients. This is not a test of your knowledge, but rather your ability to apply it appropriately. The topics will be taken from areas with which a Foundation Programme Year 2 doctor could be expected to be familiar. There are no questions requiring a specific knowledge of general practice.

Stage 3: Selection Assessment Centre (SAC). Candidates who are successful at Stage 2 are invited to a selection centre in their allocated deanery. This involves three exercises which are observed by trained assessors. These are as follows:

1. *Patient Simulation Exercise* – This will involve a simulated patient and a situation which you should be able to deal with as a doctor with at least 18 months' postgraduate experience. It will not involve a physical examination and clinical expertise is not specifically assessed.
2. *Written Exercise* – You will be given some professional integrity questions where there are no specific right or wrong answers. You will be expected to support your answers with written explanations
3. *Group Exercise* – You will be randomly allocated to a group to carry out an exercise which will involve a group discussion; this will involve interacting with candidates who are also applying for a GP Specialty Training. The group dynamics will not be assessed.

The scores of the applicants are ranked, and the higher the ranking, the higher your chance of getting your first choice post, or any post at all.

Alternative pathways to GP training

If a doctor wants to join GP specialty training, having completed posts that are relevant to general practice, they may apply to have these posts accredited towards a Certificate of Completion of Training in general practice. If the deanery accepts the post as relevant experience, the trainee may have a shortened specialty training period and apply to ST2 or even ST3 posts, depending on their experience. Trainees from abroad, for example, may have experienced similar training to that in the UK. They can submit a structured e-portfolio of their experience to the Postgraduate Medical Education and Training Board (PMETB) who then decide whether the post can be approved and whether the candidate may receive a Statement of Eligibility for Inclusion in the GP Register. If applying for shorter training (less than 36 months in total) doctors should provide evidence (VTR2 forms or ruling from the RCGP certification unit or the PMETB) that their previous experience is accredited.

Less than full time (LTFT) training

Some trainees wish to undertake their training part-time for a number of reasons. For this, deanery approval and funding is required. Exactly the same selection process applies but you must contact your preferred deaneries directly, to discuss whether LTFT would be an option in your particular circumstances. LTFT trainees must participate in all activities carried out by the department where they work, including on-call duties in the evenings and weekends. They must be prepared to work at any time of the week and at any time of the year, in the same way as their full-time colleagues. They may, however, make local arrangements for particular fixed working patterns where these can be accommodated, without prejudicing training and continuity of service delivery.

LTFT candidates need to have a suitable reason for applying, e.g. caring for young children or dependant relatives, or for personal health reasons. In the past, most LTFT trainees have been supernumerary but, with increasing numbers of applicants, supernumerary posts are now considered unaffordable in most cases. 'Slot-sharing' is the option preferred by deaneries and hospital or primary care organisations (PCOs). Consequently, finding a suitable post may depend on another LTFT trainee being available to share the same slot. LTFT training is not an easy option and takes time to organise. It is particularly difficult for general practice training, as trainees rotate through several specialties. Deaneries will give guidance but it is the responsibility of the LTFT trainee to organise their LTFT training and it is up to the trust whether they are prepared to employ them part-time for each successive post. However, all employers must seriously consider requests to work part-time and must give good reasons if they say no.

Applying for GP training from abroad

Many doctors from abroad would like to apply for training in the UK. The best way to start is to find out if you are eligible, by contacting the General Medical Council (GMC). You will need to show evidence of your qualifications, previous experience and may need other evidence such as the PLAB. For more information visit www.nhscareers.nhs.uk/img_qa.shtml.

Returner scheme

For qualified GPs who have taken an extended break from general practice and want to restart, there are, depending on funding availability, returner schemes provided in most areas. The RCGP website provides information on how to keep up professional competencies during a period away from work. You can call the Returners Hotline on 0845 6060 345 or contact your local Director of Postgraduate Education at your postgraduate deanery to find out about Returner schemes in your area. Another good source of information is the British Medical Association (BMA).

The structure of General Practice training

General practice training currently consists of a minimum of 36 months of which between 12 and 24 months are in a general practice environment doing, on average, one out-of-hours session per month. The rest are hospital-based training posts of 3–6 months each, some of which involve specialist work in the community relevant to general practice. Sometimes, this training is longer than three years in total, as there are some four-year pilot schemes available. Four-year programmes will usually include the opportunity for you to develop a special interest area in the final year.

The combination of hospital posts to form any GP training rotation will have been approved by the deanery as providing an appropriate balance of experience relevant to a future career as a GP. If you have a specific preference to complete a particular specialty post prior to your registrar year, then contact your local Programme Directors to see if your desired combination of posts is available. The core hospital posts for GP training are known as the List A specialties (*see* Table 2.1).

Table 2.1: List A specialties

Accident and emergency medicine
Paediatrics or community paediatrics
General medicine, geriatrics, dermatology, GU medicine or rehabilitation medicine
Gynaecology or Obstetrics (often combined in one post)
Psychiatry or old age psychiatry
Palliative medicine

In particular, a candidate must complete the following combination:

i.   no less than six months in each of two of the List A specialities

OR

ii. no less than four months in each of three of List A specialities

OR

iii. no less than three months in each of four of the List A Specialties.

Twelve months is the maximum time that will be accepted in any one of the List A specialities. For example, if you have done 18 months of Medicine, only 12 months will count towards your specialist training in general practice. This is to encourage a variety of experience within the posts.

If the overall programme is balanced, the Training Board will also accept training up to a maximum of six months (or its equivalent part time) for each of the List B specialties (*see* Table 2.2).

Once an applicant is accepted onto a programme they will be asked to rank their preferences from the list of rotations available on that programme. Rotation allocations will then be made either at deanery or programme level taking into account candidates preferences and assessment scores.

Throughout the programme, each trainee is supervised by an Educational Supervisor, usually one of the GP Specialty Programme Directors (PDs). Each trainee also has an allocated Clinical Supervisor for each post, who

Table 2.2: List B specialties

Cardiology, medical oncology, clinical oncology, gastroenterology, endocrinology
and diabetes mellitus, haematology, nephrology, respiratory medicine, rheumatology,
neurology or infectious diseases
Child and adolescent psychiatry, or psychiatry of learning disability
Ophthalmology, ENT, ENT surgery, general surgery, paediatric surgery, urology, trauma
and orthopaedic surgery, or trauma orthopaedics
Intensive therapy
Public health medicine

makes sure that all posts try to deliver training to complete the RCGP competencies for trainees. For example, while in a gynaecology post, the trainee should aim to obtain key competencies, such as cervical smear or female genital examination, signed off by their clinical supervisor or a designated member of the clinical team. Through a mixture of clinical experience and organised teaching, hospital posts should allow trainees to sign off certain job-specific competencies required for GP training. Most programmes now include a six-month post spent wholly or partly in general practice in the ST1 or ST2 year. This has been in response to criticisms that GP training included too much time in hospital settings.

The third (ST3) year is normally spent entirely in general practice and is usually referred to as the GP Registrar (or GPR) year. The process of allocating trainees to training practices varies between programmes. In most cases trainees are given a list of available practices in the area. Opportunities are provided to visit practices and talk to trainers and current trainees. Some form of preference matching will then take place for both trainers and trainees. Whilst you may not get your first choice, the deanery does have an obligation to ensure a practice is available for you.

In the first few weeks of the ST3 year, the trainee becomes familiar with the practice, usually sitting in with the receptionists, nurses and doctors for a few sessions and getting to know the administrative side of the practice. After this, trainees usually start surgeries, with the luxury of half an hour appointments. One session a week will be a tutorial, which the trainee and the supervisor will agree how to run. It may be that the trainee sits in on surgeries, or has observed surgeries during this session.

Otherwise, particular subjects may be prepared and discussed. One session a week is spent at the GP half-day release. The rest of the time should be working to roughly the same timetable as their trainer. In the early weeks, every surgery will be followed by a supervision session where the trainee can discuss cases. During surgery itself, the trainee should always have their trainer or another designated GP they can call for advice or to review patients, if they are not sure about particular aspects of their patients care.

It is important to establish exactly what your rota will be at the beginning of the year. You should also check your contract is clear regarding details such as salary, annual leave and study leave entitlements. Most of your time will be spent seeing patients in clinics but you will be expected to carry out home visits when appropriate, and to take part in administrative work, just like the other doctors in the practice. In essence, this year is to prepare you for working independently as a GP. As the year progresses, your appointment times will tend to become gradually shorter, aiming for 10 minutes per patient by the end of the year. See below for a checklist of key tasks for the GP Registrar year.

ST3 Checklist
- ➤ 12 out-of-hours (OOH) sessions
- ➤ 12 Clinical Consultation Observation Tools (COT) or Clinical Evaluation Exercises (CEX)
- ➤ 12 Case-Based Discussions (CBD)
- ➤ Direct Observation of Procedural Skills (DOPS) not completed during ST1 and ST2
- ➤ Get signed off every six months by your educational supervisor (GP trainer)
- ➤ Two sets of Patient Satisfaction Questionnaires (PSQs)
- ➤ Discuss with your trainer how you want to structure tutorials
- ➤ Keep your learning log up to date
- ➤ Pass the AKT and CSA (nMRCGP)
- ➤ Become confident in managing your own patients
- ➤ See patients in 10 minutes by the end of your post
- ➤ Attend GP teaching at your base
- ➤ Get important training under your belt, such as Child Protection levels 1–3
- ➤ Ideally, do one audit

In each post you may find that your practice or your deanery ask for more than the above requirements, so this is by no means a comprehensive list, only a basic guide. This is all completed in addition to adjusting to the environment of primary care and taking on significantly greater responsibility for your patients' management. Clearly this is a busy year, but as long as you are organised and motivated, it is possible to get everything done in a timely manner.

Out of programme experience

Deaneries will consider applications for out-of-programme experience (OOP) during GP training under certain circumstances, and some may have a small menu of approved OOP posts for which trainees may apply. The aim of such interruptions must be to enable GP trainees to extend their training and enhance their skills and competencies in areas that are difficult to achieve within the present three-year programme. Normally, a maximum of 12 months out of clinical training will be considered and this must not interfere with a training year, therefore it is only really possible between ST2 and ST3. Only a few deaneries organise such posts. For example, the London Deanery has offered trainees a one-year out-of-programme experience in South Africa. In some cases, if a trainee can organise an out-of-programme experience themselves, demonstrating that the post will be clinically or academically relevant to general practice, this may be approved following discussion with the deanery.

The GP educational programme

Throughout the three years of training, all GP trainees must take part in their GP educational programme (*see* Chapter 7: Professional Development for further discussion). This is often organised as one half day per week (hence known as 'half day release') but the arrangement may vary, e.g. some programmes run for one day each fortnight. Content is often negotiated and even arranged by members of the trainee group. The 'half day release' is a great way to get to know what is happening in general practice in your area, meet your fellow trainees and to socialise. This is sometimes the most important aspect for a trainee who may have a busy rota, be socially isolated in a post or have difficulties in their job that they may wish to share with other trainees or their supervisor. Practical advice about particular placements can often be obtained from trainees who have recently completed the post.

The educational programme will be facilitated by one or more Programme Directors (formerly known as Course Organisers) and sessions usually incorporate a variety of learning methods including case discussions; topic-based seminars; specialist talks; discussion of recent papers or guidelines; and Balint groups. Balint groups are small group sessions supervised by a psychologist or someone trained in running a Balint group, where doctors can bring up 'problematic' patients or patients that stay in their mind, and discuss them in relation to the effect of the patient on the doctor, and vice versa. *See* Chapter 7: Professional Development and John Salinsky's reflective piece for further discussion. In addition, most GP programmes include an annual 'residential course' which is a two- or three-day course somewhere off site. Residential courses often include team-building and group exercises, as well as more academic sessions and inspirational guest speakers.

Assessment during GP training

The e-portfolio

The online portfolio or e-portfolio is a way to record all of your learning experiences as a trainee, as well as documenting the required competencies throughout the year. On the e-portfolio you can find instructions on how to use it, how many assessments and competencies you need to achieve every six months, as well as a summary of the curriculum. Each trainee has their own e-portfolio, which they use for the whole training period. It is a record of learning, and also records whether or not the nMRCGP exam has been passed.

In the e-portfolio there are curriculum statement headings. Each time a trainee enters a learning experience onto the e-portfolio, they should link the experience to a curriculum heading, for example, an ear examination should be linked to the ear, nose and throat (ENT) heading. The aim is to ensure a broad range of coverage in all of the curriculum statements by the end of your training. The aim of each entry on the e-portfolio is to show reflective learning. Each entry should demonstrate what you have learned and how it will change your practice.

In addition to these learning experiences, your case-based discussions (CBDs), clinical evaluation exercises (CEXs) and other assessments are all accessed via the e-portfolio. While it is a time consuming process, it is very important to keep the e-portfolio up-to-date, particularly when failure to show evidence of enough learning may lead to a trainee being called to speak to the deanery panel for a review of their progress at the end of the year.

At the beginning of the post, you should create your own personal development plan on the e-portfolio, record an initial meeting with your educational and clinical supervisor, and at the end of the post, record your final meeting with your educational and clinical supervisor. The supervisor has to look through the entries in the e-portfolio intermittently to check progress and if there is satisfactory evidence and progress, the supervisor may sign off the trainee at the end of the post. A trainee may be referred to a deanery panel by their supervisor when there are concerns about their progress in a post.

All in all people either love or hate the e-portfolio, but it is currently part and parcel of being a GP trainee and does provide a systematic way of recording your experience and receiving structured feedback on your training as it progresses. In the future, it is likely that all doctors will be expected to keep evidence of their learning for revalidation, so the e-portfolio is a way of getting used to this method of keeping records and reflecting on your learning (*see* Chapter 7: Professional Development for further discussion).

About the nMRCGP

Since August 2007, the nMRCGP has been required in order to obtain a CCT (Certificate of Completion of Training) in general practice, to be on the GMC GP Register and to be a member of the RCGP. The nMRCGP is a three part assessment including:

➤ Applied Knowledge Test (AKT)
➤ Clinical Skills Assessment (CSA)
➤ Workplace-Based Assessment (WPBA)

Applied Knowledge Test

The Applied Knowledge Test is a Multiple Choice Question (MCQ) exam which, because it is a computerised MCQ test, can be taken at 'driving test' centres around the country. It can be taken at any time during training, but the RCGP recommend that it is done in the final year, as there is a higher pass rate in the final year and many of the questions are specific to experience in general practice, for example, management in general practice, sick certification and other subjects. It is a three hour exam with 200 MCQ questions covering clinical medicine, critical appraisal and statistics, health informatics and administrative issues.

Clinical Skills Assessment

The Clinical Skills Assessment (CSA) can only be done during the ST3 year. Candidates attend an assessment centre, currently in Croydon, where they take part in 13 simulated consultations, with actors playing the role of patients, and examiners assessing the candidate's response to each scenario. As well as clinical management, the trainee's problem-solving skills, person-centred care and communication skills are assessed.

Workplace-Based Assessments (WPBA)

On the RCGP curriculum you will find 12 areas of professional competence. Each trainee currently has to demonstrate competence in each of these, assessed using the WPBA.

These assessments are:

➤ Case-based Discussion (CBD) – the trainee discusses cases with their assessor.

➤ Consultation Observation Tool (COT) – the trainee is observed seeing patients either in their surgery of on videos.

➤ Multi-Source Feedback (MSF) – an anonymous form is given to members of staff working with the trainee, who then feedback their experience.

➤ Patient Satisfaction Questionnaire (PSQ) – 40 questionnaires must be completed by patients and anonymously entered onto the portfolio.

➤ Direct Observation of Procedural Skills DOPS – cover skills such as venepuncture and rectal examination.

➤ Clinical Evaluation Exercise (Mini-CEX) (mainly in hospital posts) – discussion of certain aspects of the management of a patient.

➤ Clinical Supervisors Report (CSR) – at the end of a post the supervisor gives an overview of performance.

In each six-month post trainees must complete three CEXs, three CBDs, one multi-source feedback and one CSR as well as try and sign off any relevant direct observed procedures (DOPS).

A trainee's perspective

My decision to train for general practice followed what I felt was more than enough hospital experience to know that hospital posts, although fantastic for learning and for experience of that ilk, were not for me. I had had some GP experience during my foundation years, and felt my time there was more positive, with a better relationship with my peers, and more controlled working hours. I liked the idea of more patient contact and variety, rather than super-specialising and becoming deskilled in aspects of patient care I felt interested in, such as communication, psychiatry, elderly care and preventive care, all of which can be practised simultaneously in general practice, even in a single consultation itself – the challenge of which appealed. The application process was detailed and thorough, and felt far less chaotic than any application process I had done before – this also appealed to me, knowing that general practice was a well-established specialty with an active Royal College who involved and listened to their members.

ST1

The first year of general practice training for me started with six months in elderly psychiatry. I had an initial meeting with my clinical supervisor, who went through my personal development (PDP) with me. This was a list of things I personally felt I needed to achieve by the end of the post, and helped to point out areas of doubt in my training, for example, one of my PDP points was to become familiar with the many different antipsychotics and antidepressants and how to prescribe them safely.

Every Tuesday afternoon I had leave to go to the GP half-day release teaching programme, which was a great way to get to know other trainees, share ideas and tips on how to get the most out of GP training and how to use the e-portfolio (I spent a lot of time trying to get to grips with the e-portfolio – it is quite a maze at first). In addition to GP teaching, I attended teaching in my department, and every teaching experience I had, I would try to record onto my e-portfolio. It was time-consuming however and easy to forget about the portfolio while busy on the job, especially as the only junior doctor on my ward.

The clinical supervisor and educational supervisor met each trainee at six months to make sure the e-portfolios were up-to-date. It was quite common for trainees to be behind on assessments and for the six-month review to be a reminder of the importance of the e-portfolio to progression! Supervisors varied in their use of the e portfolio, as it was a relatively new tool, and sometimes supervisors and trainees were baffled by what they were supposed to do. But, by the end of the year, most trainees and supervisors were used to it.

My second six-month post was in paediatrics, during which time I had to complete my assessments for the training as I did for the previous six months. This proved difficult as the job was very busy, and finding the time between trainee and supervising registrars or consultants to fill in the online e-portfolio could sometimes be almost impossible. Often it felt embarrassing or an impingement to ask for the assessments to be completed. This post was extremely valuable for my learning, and during this time, I had a chance to complete an audit, something that I recommend trainees to try and complete at least once during their training as audit and self-audit will be encouraged as part of your career in general practice. The hospital teaching was useful, as was the half-day release. In some jobs such as this one, it can be difficult to get time off from your service commitments to attend GP teaching, and if this becomes a recurring problem, it is worth letting your training director know, so that some arrangements can be made to help. GP trainees need to attend a minimum amount of teaching in order to get signed off at the end of each year, and trainees should feel confident about ensuring their needs are met.

ST2

My third six-month job, the beginning of my ST2 year, was an Innovative Training Post (ITP) in Women's Health. This was a new concept at the time, aiming to provide experience in both general practice and a hospital specialty. As the post was new at the time, it was my responsibility to find out how best to structure the job, so I made appointments with the relevant heads of department to work out a timetable. I was supposed to work part-time in Sexual Health and part-time in the Obstetrics and Gynaecology Department. As an ITP I was not part of the on-call rota for either of these posts. Alongside the hospital departments, I also spent two days a week in general practice.

This was a unique opportunity to become used to the GP environment one last time before my registrar year. I had my own surgeries, starting with 30 minute appointments, reducing to 15 minutes by the end of the post. At the end of each surgery, I could discuss any patients with a supervising GP. I also had one session a week for teaching with my GP trainer. On the other days, I saw patients in hospital clinics. I had the option of attending the operating theatre, going to the fertility clinics and helping on the wards. I arranged this with my educational supervisors in order to get a mixture of experience. I also clerked and reviewed patients at the antenatal clinics; all of the experience being very useful for later GP work. While the experience was incredibly varied, the only downside was that I had shorter experiences in each post, making it harder to feel part of the working environment and sometimes feeling like a 'token' member of the team, supernumerary to other clinicians.

My last six-month post was in elderly care, and general medicine, so I was back onto the on-call rota, and juggling. For the first time I had a house officer, a blessing after so long without one. Medicine was an invaluable post for future general practice, and most GP trainees will have a medical job incorporated into their ST training. I was lucky to have such varied ST1–2 posts, as I know some of my colleagues did not experience posts such as psychiatry or paediatrics. However, some colleagues had posts in ENT or palliative care, and I felt these would have been equally useful for general practice. On the other hand, experience prior to entering ST1 may compensate. For example, I had completed six months of A&E as an FY2, and so was not sad to miss out on A&E in my ST years. I was able to learn about subjects I had less experience in both through courses and clinical experience in my registrar year. Some colleagues compensated for not doing paediatrics, or obstetrics and gynaecology, by completing diplomas in these subjects. This is something an individual trainee can do if they feel it would be useful for them, though the RCGP prefer trainees to focus on the MRCGP. It is important to recognise that you will never feel confident that you have all the clinical experience necessary to be a proficient GP and will always need to continue learning as part of life as a GP.

GP Registrar year

The GP Registrar year was the most challenging yet most enjoyable of my training so far. I was lucky to spend the year in a very pro-active and up-to-date practice with an excellent trainer, as well as the additional support of other staff in the practice. As with other posts, there was an induction period, which included two weeks of sitting in with my trainer, other doctors, nurses, a healthcare assistant, specialist nurses, such as diabetic specialist, and receptionists. This was vital to learn the ins and outs of the administration of the practice (where are all the forms kept? how do you make a referral using the computer? who do you send your dictated letters to? where does your paperwork go?) and also helps familiarise you with the computer system at the practice, something which, depending on your level of computer experience, can be the most difficult part of your year!

My timetable and contract were given to me, and to begin with, my surgeries were 30 minutes per patient, and had a slot at the end to discuss every patient with my trainer. This was useful again to learn how to enter data efficiently onto the computer in such a way that others could understand it, and also to learn the basics of an effective consultation, incorporating things like preventive care and opportunistic health promotion into the consultation. I had one half day a week free which was invaluable for me to spend time with my family and friends. My surgeries mirrored those of my trainer on the whole, so that I would have a point of contact if any issues arose during the surgery. If she was away, I was assigned to another doctor in the practice.

Weekly tutorials in the practice, either with my trainer or another partner, were very useful. I tried to tackle those areas of general practice in which I felt least confident. Being aware that my exams were looming, I made sure popular exam subjects were covered. In other practices, trainees organised 'observed' surgeries so that the trainer could see first-hand how the trainee works and give feedback. I also arranged a couple of sessions like this. I chose to do the AKT as soon as I could, and arranged a study group with a few other registrars, something I would recommend to everyone. We covered guidelines and presented them to each other, and later in the year practised scenarios or cases for the Clinical Skills Assessment which we all chose to do midway through the year.

As the year continued, my surgeries were brought down to 20 minutes, 15 minutes and finally to ten minute appointments. This was decreased at a pace that myself and my trainer both felt was appropriate, rather than rushing. As well as this, supervision became more trainee-centred, so I would bring up patients I had concerns about and discuss those only, rather than the entire session.

During the year, I had to complete the WPBA and arranged it so that my tutorials could be used for this purpose. I also videoed consultations, that enabled me to complete the consultation observation tools (COT), with my trainer. It is important to do these throughout the year rather than all in a rush at the end, so I made sure there were gaps in between the assessments. The same applied for my multi source feedback (MSF) assessments and patient satisfaction questionnaire (PSQ) – getting them out of the way early and at the right time for them to be meaningful (rather than too early or late in the year) meant there was less to worry about at the end of the year, which can be incredibly busy. I carried out a small audit in the practice and presented it to the team; a useful exercise in learning how to use the computer system to audit patients.

You are given ample study leave in this year, and it is important to get vital things such as Child Protection levels one and two training done. I also chose to do the theory part of the Diploma of the Faculty of Sexual and Reproductive Healthcare (DFSRH) and Telephone Consultation Skills courses, as well as other courses aimed to help pass the exams. There are many around and you can ask your deanery about those they recommend locally.

Overall the year was challenging, as learning how to consult effectively, multitask managing the paperwork and results I received daily, as well as manage the anxieties that come with particular types of of high risk patients, was very difficult to do at the same time. On the plus side, general practice proved to be a much better learning environment for me than my previous posts. I was always well supported, and felt no qualms about asking any colleagues for advice without feeling fear or embarrassment, knowing that the entire practice can learn from anything that you raise. The only downside of the year was that it felt far less sociable than my previous hospital posts. Often doctors would work through their lunch break, or you would be on a home visit or have paperwork to do which meant you couldn't meet others in the practice. This meant that the weekly half day release teaching was an extremely sociable occasion, much appreciated by all the registrars.

Juggling all the above, plus the exams, is a challenge but works out well in some ways, as you are forced to keep up-to-date on clinical issues because you are studying outside of your working day, and looking up things as you see them in clinical practice. I was given a taste of not only how much responsibility there is as a GP, but also how much support a GP can receive from their colleagues. I learnt more about my own learning styles, vital for future practice as a GP.

Overall, the GP Registrar year was the most enjoyable year of my training, representing a final satisfying hurdle, where you are expected to become ready for 'real' general practice. It is very satisfying to experience the feeling that everything you have learnt during your training has actually made a difference to your practice, as you are faced with challenges mirroring those you had in previous posts, but with the experience to handle them better. I learnt the most I ever have, in a supportive learning environment, and felt ready to continue to learn and change when I left.

Conclusion

In this chapter, we have briefly outlined the history of specialty GP training, the process of applying for training, the structure of the training programme and assessment procedures along the way. GP training is now a highly structured, monitored and assessed process. This is necessary to ensure fair selection, appropriate quality of supervision and training as well as adequate competence before entering independent practice. The various hoops and hurdles should be easily managed by any enthusiastic and motivated trainee. There is guidance available along the way and the experience of GP training, while sometimes challenging and demanding, should always be interesting and prepare trainees to become lifelong learners. There is no way a trainee can learn everything in their three years of training, and so, a trainee should be prepared to keep up-to-date and use their learning skills to do so throughout their career.

Reference

Tooke J. *Aspiring to Excellence, Final Report of the Independent Inquiry into Modernising Medical Careers;* 2008. [Online]. Available at: www.mmcinquiry.org.uk/draft.htm (accessed 25 July 2010).

Useful resources

Applying from abroad visit www.nhscareers.nhs.uk/img_qa.shtml

BMJ Careers www.bmjcareers.com

Emedica online revision – interactive revision for stage 2 MCQ assessment www.emedica.co.uk/mcqs.htm

A list of all UK Deaneries can be found at www.gprecruitment.org.uk/deaneries.htm

London Deanery provide details of all training schemes and training practices in the London area www.londondeanery.ac.uk/general-practice/specialty-training-for-gp

General Medical Council www.gmc-uk.org

Modernising Medical Careers (MMC) www.mmc.nhs.uk

National Recruitment Office for General Practice Training www.gprecruitment.org.uk

The Royal College of General Practitioners (RCGP) provides detailed advice on GP training and also certification via www.rcgp.org.uk/gp_training.aspx www.rcgp.org.uk/certification_/certification_home.aspx
RCGP curriculum www.rcgp-curriculum.org.uk
Free articles and advice on the application process, ST2 and ST3 assessments and GP training in the UK www.gpvts.info

Reflective piece: 'Medical maternal'

Anne Solomon

I came late to medicine. After a short career as a classical violinist, I was almost thirty before I started medical school. I continued as an occasional jobbing musician up until I reached my house jobs, when the onerous hours forced me to put every other interest in my life to one side. I took a year out to recuperative after that, to propose to my boyfriend (who generously forgave my stroppy, sleep-deprived behaviour of the previous year) and also complete a recording contract for some obscure but beautiful sonatas by the Romanian composer George Enescu. Halfway through this year, I fell pregnant and married. Life became a jumble of rich possibilities and clashing demands.

Enter the flexible training office (FTO); the deanery department which organises part-time postgraduate training. It agreed to finance my GP training as long as I could secure a job 'in open competition'. That meant applying for posts, somewhat covertly, as a full-timer. The FTO stepped in to create the part-time package if and when you got the job. This was done either by finding another trainee to job share with, or creating a new 'supernumerary' part-time post, fully funded by the FTO. Job shares were much cheaper for them, but it was hard to find another doctor to share with, so most of my training was supernumerary. Organising these supernumerary posts was largely up to me and often involved a colossal amount of time communicating with the various medical training bodies and personnel. On the other hand, this process allowed me to tailor my education to my learning needs in a way no full-time trainee could dream of.

Two pieces of good luck helped me through my training: being funded by the FTO, and being accepted by my local GP training scheme. Without these, I doubt I would ever have made it through. It is tough being a mother of young children in medicine. The profession is famously unsupportive of doctors' needs, and this is so culturally entrenched that flexible trainees are sometimes regarded as pampered by their colleagues, whereas in fact they are struggling every step of the way to hold job and family together.

I began my GP training with a six-month old baby and will never forget the indignity of expressing milk in the NHS toilets during my lunch break – it was the only privacy I could find. I was heavily pregnant with my second during psychiatry and felt vulnerable on the acute ward, where I feared the most psychotic patients might weave my pregnancy into their delusions. By the end of my registrar training I had three children under six.

At work, I often felt set apart from the other trainees. This was partly because I was older than most of them. In addition I was part-time, supernumerary and often not directly involved with the on-call rota, and this distanced me from the herd. Whilst privileged to avoid some of the dross, I envied what I perceived as their casual comradeship. I saw myself as the bumbling part-timer who was never quite confident with the job, or with trainee culture, who was always rushing off apologetically, soon after 5pm, to pick up children from nursery. This excuse sounded lame to my ears, like a soldier downing his gun mid-battle to attend to some housework. Tearing through London traffic, to reach the nursery before it closed, was another regular sufferance. Then there was the husband who was left literally holding the baby whenever I was working late. Life was a perpetual round of apologies.

I have no regrets about training part-time. I was lucky enough to be taken on before the FTO lost funding and then had to turn many mothers away. Some of these stuck it out as full-time trainees with the unstinting support of partners and extended families. I met a few along the way and their lives sounded far more difficult than mine. Others, I am sure, quit medicine as a result, unable to marry the needs of their children with their careers.

The pitfall of part-time training is its disjointed nature, which can prevent one from gaining fluency. I chose to work at 60% full-time (the minimum allowed at that time) giving me a three-day working week. My GP training, including maternity leave, took me six years to complete instead of three. On the other hand, because my posts lasted longer I saw more pathology pass through the wards. The continuity I lost at work I gained with my children, which many mums working full-time miss out on.

Looking back at my traineeship, at its worst I was tired and strained by the demands of career and young family. At best, I went to work with zest and returned to my kids with joy. I would not say my work-life balance was perfect, but it came pretty close at times.

Reflective piece: 'Extraordinary ordinary people'

Alex Thain

I am an ordinary GP in an ordinary surgery in the North of Scotland and I feel privileged. Why privileged, you may ask…? Well, I have the good fortune to meet and work with some special people.

I'd start with Jean. I suppose that I had always known in a subliminal way that she was special but it was only when discussing her husband's death that her abilities actually penetrated my consciousness. Bill had a vicious, progressive neurological disease and probably had not recognised her for years. She had the sad misfortune of two bereavements. The second was easier to pinpoint, Bill's final and definite physical death was shrouded in sadness but released them both. The first was an intermittent, slow and lingering bereavement, as she gradually lost the man she'd married and had children with. It was vague and nebulous, flitting between the clouds of diagnosis, realisation and acceptance. I have been genuinely humbled by her reserves of capability and oceans of emotional warmth packaged in a skin of modesty and practicality. Her insights into the difficult decisions surrounding Bill's care were a virtual textbook of ethics which she referenced innately and instinctively, always keeping his interests to the fore, despite the costs to herself. Jean sought neither gain nor recognition and I admire her immensely.

I'd probably introduce Jimmy next. He's the stalwart head of a complex fractured modern family and was, technically, the Grandpa but effectively the father of the youngster who died. A child's death is always traumatic and ripples from the event's impact on families, friends, professionals and communities. I spent a great deal of time with the family at this intimate time and witnessed grief, care, wisdom and philosophy flourishing within the walls of that small terraced house in a sprawling council scheme. After the funeral, the family were facing their next phase, accepting that life would return to normal for others in just a few days, whilst their life had changed irrevocably. I was outside with Jimmy, chatting as we surveyed the neighbours working in their gardens. Jimmy paused, looked straight ahead and said slowly 'Aye Doc, grass still grows while you grieve'. The clarity, simplicity and insight of the metaphor were as stunning as they were unexpected. The insight had shades of TS Eliot and the alliteration rhythm and scan would pass for Auden, yet the words simply reflected how he felt. Jimmy has a basic education and could not begin to conceive of himself as a poet or a philosopher, but that's how I see him.

Alexandra's situation is a familiar one: a difficult childhood evolving into an adolescence of drug misuse crystallising into an adulthood of chronically low self-esteem reinforced by her financial and housing problems. And yet, at an ordinary party in an ordinary flat someone collapsed and stopped breathing. Nothing happened. The great and good, the capable and confident, the sober and inebriated stood and looked. Only Alexandra was prepared to take any responsibility and commenced resuscitation. She did it on her own at first and then with telephone guidance from our Ambulance colleagues. Unfortunately, the patient did not survive, nor was he ever going to, but predictably Alexandra struggles to move beyond her perception of failure. I hope that in time she can see the strength and courage of her actions. I'm probably not supposed to be proud of her, the doctor-patient relationship shouldn't be like that, but as a human being I'm immensely proud of her.

These tales offer a glimpse of the many, many individuals who have shared their emotions and insights with me. I've changed their names and mixed up their stories to protect their confidentiality, but the events are real.

I am an ordinary GP, in an ordinary surgery, in the North of Scotland and I *am* privileged.

CHAPTER 3

Salaried jobs and partnerships

Judith Harvey

Since the founding of the NHS in 1948, most GPs have been independent contractors: self-employed doctors who have entered into a contract with the management of the NHS to provide general medical services for NHS patients. The majority of independent contractors work in partnerships; some are single-handed. A sizeable minority of GPs are employed on a salary. A third group of GPs work as locums (*see* Chapter 4: Locum and out-of-hours work). This chapter looks at partnership and salaried jobs.

The working lives of GPs in the twenty-first century are very different from those of family doctors in the 1950s. Now, nearly half of general practitioners are women. Then, the term 'work-life balance' was unknown; now doctors of both sexes expect to have a life outside their primary job and more variety within it. Government policy and societal changes affect the balance between the number of GPs and the employment opportunities. Some years you can take your pick of jobs; at other times you may be one of hundreds of applicants applying for each vacancy that is advertised.

How GPs work within the NHS

As you come to the end of your registrar (ST3) year, what sort of employment opportunities will be available and which might suit you best? Understanding the options will help direct your search.

Independent contractors

Independent GP contractors, known until 2004 as 'principals' and now as 'providers', are GPs who contract with a Primary Care Organisation (PCO) to provide primary healthcare services for a local population. They are often called 'partners' as shorthand, although around 6% of providers are single-handed. Providers are self-employed and, within limits set by their contract with the PCO, are free to organise the provision of services as they see fit.

Practices either have a nationally negotiated contract to provide General Medical Services (GMS), or a locally negotiated contract to provide Personal Medical Services (PMS). PMS contracts were introduced in 1998 to offer local flexibility: where GPs were hard to recruit, nurses could hold contracts, and remuneration could be structured to reward practices for good care of groups such as the homeless, whose needs were not adequately recognised by the GMS contract. In 2004, much of that flexibility was introduced into the new national GMS contract, and now PMS are usually closely modelled on the GMS contract. The basic income for standard medical services which all practices must provide is based on the number of patients registered with the practice, and can be supplemented by provision of a range of 'enhanced' services. Extra income can be earned through the Quality and Outcomes Framework (QOF), which offers additional money for good clinical and managerial practice.

The Alternative Provider Medical Services (APMS) contract, introduced in 2005, enables PCOs to contract with private non-NHS management organisations. These may be GP practices, charities or private organisations. The contract is very flexible: contractors can subcontract the provision of services, contracts can be of short duration and be for only parts of the service. Additionally, PCOs now directly employ some GPs, either to provide full general practice services or to take advantage of a GPs special skills to provide a particular service for all patients in a locality (*see* Chapter 5: GPs with a specialist interest).

Salaried (employed) GPs

Until 2004, the term 'non-principals' was used to distinguish all salaried and locum GPs from 'principals'. The terms 'sessional GP' and 'freelance GP' are now generally used to describe any GP who is not an independent contractor, although 'sessional' is sometimes equated with 'salaried' and 'freelance' with locum. A GP partner or employed GP may also do locum sessions, and GPs of all categories can work for out-of-hours services.

Salaried GPs may be employed by practices, PCOs or APMS organisations. In the days when partnership was the norm, salaried GPs were a small and sometimes exploited minority. At the time of writing, economic factors encourage practices to employ GPs rather than appoint partners. Since 2004, PCOs contract with practices rather than individual doctors, so GPs no longer have their own lists of patients, and now many patients of both GP partnerships and APMS practices receive their care from teams of salaried GPs. It is not unusual now for GPs to be salaried for part or all of their professional lives.

Most salaried posts are fully funded by the employing practice. However, when there is a shortage of GPs, governments may seek to maintain the workforce by subsidising practices to employ part-time GPs who might oth-erwise 'drop out', providing them with some degree of education support or mentoring. Such posts have often proved so popular that the schemes have been withdrawn once the manpower crises they were introduced to amelio-rate are resolved. Nevertheless, funding for the oldest scheme, the Retainer Scheme, is generally still available (BMA, 2007b).

There are standard contracts for subsidised schemes. Because GPs employed in unsubsidised posts are more exposed to the marketplace, the British Medical Association (BMA) developed a model contract to protect them (BMA, 2009). The good terms and conditions, particularly for study leave, reflect the fact that in 2004, when the contract was devised, demand for salaried GPs exceeded supply. Its use is mandatory for GMS practices and it is recommended to all other employers. However, many practices claim that, as the NHS belt has tightened, they cannot afford such generous terms, and some GMS practices even compensate themselves by demanding a very high workload in return for a low salary. Private providers, despite the prejudice against them, are sometimes better employers than traditional GP practices. If you are considering a salaried post, you should study the contract you are offered very carefully and if its terms appear substandard be prepared to negotiate, and seek advice if necessary. The BMA's *Salaried GPs' Handbook*, a comprehensive guide to salaried posts, is available on-line to BMA members (BMA, 2010).

The income of salaried doctors is almost always less than that of partners. This reflects the fact that it is generally, though not always, a buyer's market. Also, partners, unlike employed GPs, have responsibility for their practices and this is recognised in their remuneration.

Salaried roles in general practice are evolving. Out-of-Hours (OOH) pro-viders employ GPs. For some GPs, this accounts for most or all of their income. GPs are also employed to provide primary care services for social groups poorly served by traditional general practice, such as travellers. There are also posts within the NHS for GPs with special skills such as sports medi-cine. In the commercial world, GPs are in demand: from ship's doctor (*see* Chapter 9: International Primary Care) to advisor to medical soap operas; the opportunities are there if you keep looking.

Locums

Locums are self-employed GPs who offer their services on a freelance basis to fill manpower gaps which are usually short-term, but can last several months or even years. (*See* Chapter 4 for more about locum work).

Making your choice: what sort of GP do you want to be?

In the 1970s 'A Fortunate Man', John Berger's lyrical photojournalistic essay about the life and work – the two almost indistinguishable – of John Sassall, a single-handed rural GP, shaped the aspirations of a generation of idealistic doctors (Berger, 1967). The world has changed, but most GPs still hope that their career will be touched by the magic that emanates from the pages of Berger's book, and they see independent contractor status as the route through which the dream is most likely to be realised. Others, perhaps remembering that Sassall later committed suicide, may wonder if that identification with the pain of patients' lives was bought at too high a cost, and look to a career where work and life outside it are more balanced.

Partnership: pros and cons

As an independent contractor, whether single-handed or in partnership, you make a long-term commitment to your practice, and to the community it serves. You can look forward to a lifetime of investment and reward. You have as much control as the government allows over the way you work: you can shape the way you provide services to suit your patients and your own ambitions and needs. You can become part of the community. You are able to develop shared projects with other local organisations. You can expect good financial rewards. Your spouse can take work knowing that you are both committed to the area; your children can stay at the same school and with the same friends; you can nurture social and leisure networks.

The intangible rewards have not changed much over the years, but the practicalities have. In 1948, most GPs worked alone. In 1965, a crisis of morale in general practice resulted in the Family Doctors' Charter (RBLMC, 2010). This set the structure for the modern NHS by providing money for investment in premises, staff, GP education and new services. Many GPs saw the advantages of joining together in group practices. Now, most GPs work in partnerships. As a partner, you can expect to develop your own interests, whether they are clinical or business, and to be spared, to some degree, the aspects of the job you are less suited to.

Income depends on profits and is not guaranteed, but GP partners are generally high earners. Most partnerships share the profits; a few pay all partners a salary. New partners usually have to buy into a share of the practice's assets. If the practice owns its own premises, this may involve substantial financial investment. Loans are usually available for what has traditionally been a very good investment, so the cost of 'buying in' is unlikely to stand between you and a partnership.

Partnerships vary in their ethos. Partners in a harmonious partnership usually share, to some degree, a motivation or ideal, be it social, political or religious. This may be overt and advertisements for new partners will make clear the practice's wish to recruit someone with the same views. Other practices share a general philosophy of patient care, but otherwise do not concern themselves with their colleagues' beliefs, as long as these do not impinge on the practice.

However, shared visions are not a guarantee of permanent harmony. A degree of difference is generally constructive: the grit in the oyster shell which gives rise to the pearl. Partnership is a team and partners need to be team players: able to negotiate, compromise, and to accept being outvoted – sometimes on matters about which they care deeply.

In the olden days, a GP tucked his legs – and they were almost invariably in trousers – under a consulting room desk in his mid-twenties and didn't move until the day when hundreds of grateful patients queued up to wish him a happy retirement. GPs still enter a partnership with the expectation that it will be long term, but now moving to a new partnership is accepted. If your spouse gains a consultant post 500 miles away or if you are stuck in a dead-end practice, you can move on. Even a refugee from an acrimonious partnership split is not an outcast: sadder, possibly poorer, hopefully wiser, but not ruled out of future short lists.

Partnerships, like marriages and cars, need regular servicing. Partnership meetings facilitate day-to-day smooth running, away-days are useful for tackling strategic challenges and occasional social events lubricate relationships. But if profound differences arise, it is important to have an agreed mechanism for resolving the situation. It is not unusual for partnerships to become divided: one partner or group of partners is consistently outvoted by the majority. Once this situation is entrenched, it is hard to resolve except by dissolving the partnership so that both sides can go their separate ways, hopefully amicably. Practices must be prepared for a bitter divorce, and your practice agreement should include clauses which, like pre-nuptial agreements, state the terms which determine the end of the partnership.

Single-handed practice: pros and cons

If you find your ambitions cramped in a partnership, you may consider going single-handed to realise your vision, unfettered by partners who are not prepared to change.

Governments do not like single-handed practices. Patients do. Governments remember the days of isolated doctors practising poor quality medicine out of lock-up premises with no form of education or audit. They have not forgotten that Dr Harold Shipman, convicted in 2000 of murdering his patients, was a single-hander. Patients, however, consistently show high satisfaction with single-handed practices, valuing the personal relationship between patient and GP and the continuity of care they receive (Baker, 1995).

Being single-handed requires determination and sacrifice, but for the right person – likely to be a self-starting individualist with a very clear vision – it is intensely rewarding. Many single-handers continue doing their own on-call work: they know their patients, their patients respect them and will only call in a real emergency. But if you are considering working single-handed you must bear in mind that you are ultimately responsible for absolutely everything, whether you are consulting in Cheltenham or lazing in Lanzarote. It can be difficult to set up cover arrangements which allow a single-hander to take time off to relax, confident that the practice is in safe hands. You need to be resourceful, able to cope alone with crises, and be pro-active (though a good practice manager makes a huge contribution). You do not have partners who can cover if you are ill, so a robust physical and mental constitution is essential. An understanding spouse is invaluable, especially as such a strong tie to the practice can be hard for families.

While it is possible to sustain a single-handed practice in isolation, co-operative working with other practices can be advantageous. This offers opportunities to share services, skills, education and staff for whom a practice does not have a full-time requirement, as well as providing cross-cover and commissioning services.

Because of official concerns about their standards, single-handers have to constantly be able to demonstrate their cost-effectiveness, their financial and clinical probity, their robust clinical governance and their patients' satisfaction.

When single handed practices become vacant, PCOs usually take them over and either merge them with existing practices or install alternative providers. Therefore, the General Practitioners Committee (GPC) of the BMA advises single-handers approaching retirement, who want to preserve their practices, to take on a partner to hand the practice over to (BMA, 2007a). If you are considering single-handed practice, working as an employed GP to a single hander with a view to inheriting the practice allows you to get to know the patients and the practice's strengths (and weaknesses) and to take over smoothly when the time comes.

Salaried pros and cons

A salaried post offers a job description and a guaranteed income. Salaried GPs do not own the business in which they work, so do not have the responsibility of managing it, nor, unlike locums, do they have to manage their own business.

A salaried post may appeal because you want to concentrate on seeing patients. If you are either at the beginning or end of your career you may be happy to be free from the responsibility of the finances, building, staff, policies, organisation and all the other burdens of the practice where you work.

A salaried post may suit your domestic situation or health. You may only be able to commit a few years to one place, or have a portfolio career but still want to maintain your general practice skills. You may take a salaried job because partnerships are not available, or because you hope that a spell in a practice as a salaried GP may lead to a partnership.

The right salaried post – in a practice of like-minded colleagues who offer good terms and conditions and treat employees as valued team members – is like a well-fitting shoe. However, a post in the wrong practice can rub you raw. To some extent, areas of friction can be anticipated and if you are considering taking a salaried post you need to examine the potential problem areas.

An employee with a very different style of practice from the partners is likely to be uncomfortable. For instance, if partners bring patients back for review much more frequently than you (or *vice versa*) there can be friction over how the workload is shared. You will have to fit in with the practice's clinical policies. In some APMS practices these may be rigidly determined. Taking time to find out in advance whether you will be comfortable in the practice is a good investment. Asking crucial questions at interview is important. A few days working as a locum can provide the definitive answer.

Common problems that you must clarify before you sign a contract include unrealistic workloads in face-to-face consultation as well as administrative tasks, lack of opportunities for study leave and continuing professional development (CPD), poor pay and unfair conditions. Unfortunately, some practices do not honour the signed contract, and a few expect their employees to work before agreeing a contract. You need to have the confidence to demand the BMA model contract from GMS practices and to expect it from PMS and APMS practices, and to seek help if you think you are being unfairly treated.

Attending practice meetings can often be a sore point. For part-timers, whether partners or salaried, attending meetings can be very difficult due to other commitments. But not being at such meetings excludes you from information, education and involvement. Good practices will be open to negotiation on what meetings are regarded as essential (and therefore happen in paid time). Aim to attend as many meetings as possible which deal with clinical governance and policy, for example, significant event audits and clinical reviews. If you cannot attend, circulation of agendas and minutes helps to keep you in touch.

Not all practices make employed doctors feel like second-class citizens! Good practices will offer their salaried GPs opportunities to become involved in special projects and to take on responsibilities in the practice, and engaged employees will be keen to offer their services, to take up opportunities, and to go out of their way to help their practice. (If a partnership becomes vacant within the practice, salaried doctors who do this will be the first to be considered, and those who provided the minimum contractual service will not find themselves shortlisted.) But if you are an employee, you have to accept that you are working in someone else's business. You may be encouraged to contribute to decision-making debates, but ultimately you are not responsible for the practice. Often it is the desire to have more control which propels GPs into seeking a partnership.

If salaried status suits you, you have to bear in mind that you are unlikely to have a job for life. When your contract comes to an end, the job market may have changed. There may be more opportunities, but there could also be fewer. As a salaried GP, you have to be prepared to rethink your career and to see this as an opportunity, not a threat.

Is partnership for me?

Any job is what you make it, but the scope depends on the team around you. There are congenial and irritating partners as well as supportive and exploitative employers.

Your expectations of partnership need to be realistic. It is never going to be plain sailing all the way. Be prepared for difficult times. A mistake some young GPs make is expecting that partners will also be friends. Essentially, it is a business relationship and few GPs expect to spend their leisure time with their professional partners.

Most registrars are very happy at their training practice, and becoming a partner there can offer the expectation of a lifetime of professional satisfaction. Sadly, such dreams can turn to nightmares. Being a registrar and being a partner are very different. Wonderful trainers can prove infuriating business partners. Practice managers who are splendidly supportive to registrars can reveal themselves as unable to handle staff conflicts or disastrous at maintaining financial control. The receptionist who used to indulge you as a registrar may find it hard to accept being disciplined by you when you become a partner.

Any newly qualified GP is well advised to spend some time working in several different practices to experience other ways of doing things. If you are considering a partnership at your training practice a break between registrar and partner status is particularly valuable. Working as a locum in the practice can show the partners, the staff, and their ethos in a different light. Working at other practices can be invaluable experience and the time out will make the change in status easier to navigate.

If you have applied for a partnership, how do you decide if it is for you? You have considered all the points discussed in this chapter. You have checked the accounts and the local schools, the partners say they will encourage you to become a trainer and would exploit your experience in acupuncture, you and the practice manager share a passion for bird watching, and the team meet every morning over a cup of good coffee. What else will help you decide? Will the personality profiling help? How much will trial by dinner at the senior partner's home tell you? Will taking a surgery or a spell as a locum reveal valuable clues? The answer is, all of these will give you more information but ultimately, you must trust your own judgement. And once a partner be prepared to be flexible. Practices and people – including you – change with time. If you are lucky, you and the practice will grow together. If you are unlucky, and decide the only way out is resignation, the experience you will take with you will be invaluable.

Combining personal and professional partnership

GP couples can find the combination of a professional and personal partnership tempting. It avoids the conflict of interest which can arise when couples work in rival practices, and it can be very constructive and rewarding. But if you are a GP couple considering practising together, it is worth anticipating any possible problems.

Like a single-hander, you may find it difficult to arrange cover that you trust sufficiently to allow you to take holidays. It is also worth considering how you would manage the introduction of a third partner. Anyone joining an established husband-and-wife team risks always being outvoted or being pig in the middle. And a rocky period in either the professional or the marital partnership can easily put the other relationship under strain. Partnership break-up is always traumatic and so is divorce; to go through both at the same time, with the same person on the other side of both conflicts can be devastating. Still, for the right couple, combining professional and personal partnership can be very satisfying.

The crystal ball

It is not easy to forecast the future shape of careers in general practice. Many pressures affect the job opportunities open to GPs. Governments are trying to manage both the GP workforce and individual GPs practice ever more closely, and there is no doubt that it is easier to control the costs and work of salaried doctors than independent contractors. It is unclear, at the time of writing, how the introduction of practice-based commissioning will affect the job market. However, the survival of the independent contractor status is not just determined by governments; it also depends on GPs. Currently many practices are advertising for salaried GPs rather than partners. But if GPs want partnerships, and if practices are encouraged to appoint them, partnerships will survive. And if you do not want a partnership, a search through the advertisements for salaried posts may reveal the ideal post for you. Whatever the job market is when you come to look for work, the more you understand about the opportunities and limitations inherent in the post you apply for, the more satisfied you are likely to be with the job when you are successful.

References

Baker R, Streatfield J. What type of general practice do patients prefer?: Exploration of practice characteristics influencing patient satisfaction. *Brit J Gen Pract.* 1995; **45**: 654–659.

Berger J. *A Fortunate Man: Story of a Country Doctor.* London: Penguin; 1967.

BMA. *Contractual Issues for GPs;* 2007a. [Online]. Available at: www.bma.org. uk/employmentandcontracts/independent_contractors/providing_gp_ services/contractissuesgps0407.jsp (accessed 7 June 2010).

BMA. *Model GP retainer scheme contract;* 2007b [Online]. Available at: www. bma.org.uk/employmentandcontracts/employmentcontracts/salaried_gps/ contractretainerGP.jsp (accessed 7 June 2010).

BMA. *Model salaried GP contract: GMS practice;* 2009. [Online]. Available at: www.bma.org.uk/employmentandcontracts/employmentcontracts/ salaried_gps/SalariedGPcontractGMS0209.jsp (accessed 7 June 2010).

BMA. *Salaried GPs' handbook: A guide for salaried GPs and their employers;* 2010. [Online]. Available at: www.bma.org.uk/employmentandcontracts/ employmentcontracts/salaried_gps/salariedgpbook.jsp (accessed 7 June 2010).

RBLMC. *The History of Local Medical Committees;* 2010. [Online]. Available at: www.randblmc.nhs.uk/lmc-history.html (accessed 7 June 2010).

Career profile:

Clifton Marks

When did you qualify

MB BS, University of London, Middlesex Hospital Medical School 1982. Subsequently DRCOG , and MRCGP – which I took in 1995 at the same time as training my first registrar. I completed GP training in 1987 which did not require MRCGP at that time.

What is your job?

I am a partner in a large inner city general practice. The practice services a culturally diverse population, which includes one of the largest Chassidic communities in Europe.

Why and how did you choose General Practice?

I more or less decided while at medical school. As I rotated through the various specialities, although I found some more interesting than others, I realised I could not spend my entire career specialising in one part of the body. I strongly believed in looking after the whole person. I also found that the hospital was a very dehumanising environment, and preferred the autonomy and 'real world' of the community. This was reinforced by what was then called the 'trainee year' now ST3. I was fortunate to train in a lovely practice and with an inspiring trainer.

Where did you work?

Initially I did house jobs (now FY1) in St Albans and Staffordshire, followed by posts in Dermatology, Medicine for the Elderly, Obstetrics and Gynaecology and Accident and Emergency Medicine (A&E). A&E was very useful as it trained me to assess patients very quickly and included extreme hospital emergencies as well as general practice cases presenting inappropriately to A&E. It also included paediatrics. The rest of paediatrics and GP orientated psychiatry was learned in the general practice year. I had decided for personal and family reasons that I wanted to stay in North London, which dictated my choice of practice. I always wanted to work in a large practice which was involved in teaching and owned its own premises.

After finishing GP training, I locumed for a year which was also useful gaining experience before joining my present practice in 1988. During the locum year I became involved in reproductive health, doing sessions at the Margaret Pyke Centre, and later worked as a sessional doctor with what eventually became Enfield Primary Care Trust (PCT). I later become an

Associate Specialist doing one session a week in addition to my general practice commitment.

In 1993 I became a trainer replacing one of my senior partners who was retiring. In 1999 after the retirement of the senior partner I became the 'financial partner' of the practice. This is not everyone's cup of tea but modern general practice is a business perhaps even more so now than ever before. Also at the end of the 1990s I was elected to the Local Medical Committee (LMC). As we were such a large practice there was a tradition of someone being on the LMC, as it allowed us to get a feel for what was going on politically.

What is the most rewarding aspect of your job?
Providing personal medical care to patients you can actually help. It can be very frustrating at times as many patients have problems which cannot be solved. When you are able to make a difference it's very rewarding, whether this is *just* listening to people or making a more traditional diagnosis. I also like helping trainees. I am fortunate in working within a stable mutually supportive partnership. I also value the good relationships I have with colleagues.

What is the most challenging or frustrating aspect of your job?
Never having enough time. One is always left with the feeling your work is never finished, which is coupled with the increasing encroachment of over-regulation and bureaucracy.

If you could change one thing about your career, what would it be?
Apart from my student elective in the USA, I have never worked abroad.

What do you wish you knew then that you know now?
The importance of communication, whether it is with patients or colleagues. Although I always knew this was important I now realise it is *really* important. You must look after yourself as well. Never be afraid to ask for help if you think you need it. There is only one way to get experience and it takes time.

Reflective piece: 'Good enough'

Rebecca Ship

I meet Mrs K. in town one cold weekday about six months after I've left the practice – bundled up in her coat and scarf and, standing at a bus stop, looking tired. As I approach, she squints against the weak winter sun behind me, and then, recognising me, she smiles. I'm struck by the warmth of that smile, the way it seems to relieve her face of its wrinkled tension. She greets me, and when I ask her how she is, she tightens, and the smile fades, and then quickly returns. She gives her usual stoical response, and berates me gently for leaving when I did. Not that she begrudges me my retirement, but you know things aren't the same now, the practice is so huge, she can't keep up with all the changes, and she doesn't really know any of the doctors now – they're so young. Don't get me wrong, she says, they're very good, but it's not the same, is it? There is a pause, while I contemplate this. I'm not quite sure what to say in response. No, it certainly is not quite the same, and hasn't been for a long time. This is one of the reasons I left, deciding to retire a year early. I cannot begin to explain the complicated surge of emotions I experience when I try to make sense of my actions. It all seems so long ago – the sense of weariness, the waves of what I called paper-panic that threatened to swamp me if I relaxed my vigilance, the strange combination of fear and boredom which confused and exhausted me every day.

And yet, and yet … there was laughter, too, with patients and with colleagues, and kindness, and those moments when knowledge and intuition collide in a thoroughly gratifying way – a blood test that clarifies an ambiguous clinical picture, a referral that gets results, a treatment that works – that sort of thing. What do I have to complain about? It was a good job, satisfying in a way I know I'm privileged to have experienced. If it sometimes smacked of routine and tedium and trivia, the compensation was in the possibility of something unexpected happening – which it did, quite often.

I don't miss it, though. In the early days, I would wake in the morning with a frisson of anxiety tugging at my innards. What is it I have to do today? Ah, yes – nothing. It was rather unnerving, at first, to have all that unstructured time in front of me. I could make plans, fantasise or simply 'be'. This is quite hard when you are used to timetables and a heavily circumscribed day, measured in 10 minute chunks and always, always running late. Now, everything is wide open. With the shedding of responsibility for other lives comes permission to – well, to choose to do as little or as much as I want, as superficially or intensely as I want, and to spend as much or as little time as I want doing whatever it is I've chosen to do. And if I can no longer boast a rather nebulous sense of professional pride, it has been replaced by the comforting knowledge that I am accountable only to myself. I still want to do well, but at least I don't have to have a licence to practise.

I am occasionally taken aback by the reactions of ex-patients I run into. The fierceness of their gratitude is humbling. I think about what kind of a doctor I was. Did I pay enough attention? Was I careless in some way? I remember Mrs K. smiling bleakly at the bus stop and I think that, on the whole, I was probably good enough.

CHAPTER 4

Locum and out-of-hours work

Jennifer Chodera

Overview

This chapter outlines what working as a locum or out-of-hours (OOH) doctor might entail, aiming to give a flavour to help you decide whether this style of working could suit you. Towards the end of the chapter is some practical advice: firstly how to get started, then how to continue developing yourself and your career.

Both locum and OOH general practice work involve providing primary medical care for patients when their own GP is unavailable. The responsibility of the doctor in both situations is to provide good, safe medical care on that day, and to provide any necessary safety-netting and handover. The locum GP sees the patient within normal working hours in the practice where the patient is registered, which may include a variety of settings e.g. prison, young offender institutions or military bases both in the UK and abroad. OOH care is also provided in a variety of settings once the surgery is closed, including A&E, Minor Injuries Units, Walk-in Centres or Primary Care Centres. The OOH period varies within England, Scotland and Wales, but is currently from around 6.00–6.30pm to 8.00am on weekdays (plus some additional afternoons for a few smaller practices) and 24 hours a day during weekends and bank holidays.

Both types of work are most often based on shorter-term contracts, which can be anything from a session upwards, but sometimes a locum or OOH doctor can have long-term regular work within one setting and, therefore, be a fully participating member of the team.

Both locum and OOH work allow one to develop a portfolio career. Some GPs develop a lifelong career as a locum or OOH doctor, and hopefully as this chapter develops, you will see why this can be a positive personal career choice.

Historical changes

Even just a few decades ago, locums made up a tiny proportion of the general practice workforce, but now represent one-quarter of all GPs. Although until the 1990s almost the only career option for GPs was to become a partner, there is now greater variety in employment opportunities, reflecting the more complex provision of primary care. There are moves to further profes-sionalise the status of the locum GP, who historically has been perceived to be a 'lesser' doctor. There are now groups of locum doctors coming together to form 'locum chambers', where staff are employed to manage administra-tion, an education programme and clinical meetings. Chambers may even offer feedback to employing practices, illustrating the increasing acknowl-edgment and value of a two-way relationship between practices and locums.

It is fitting that the role of locum GPs be acknowledged and further valued, as they have a crucial role in the delivery of high quality primary care. Whereas in the past, there were no computer systems to grapple with, and referring would have been by a more or less standard procedure, nowa-days, the locum needs to adapt to computer systems as well as a variety of surgeries, different patient populations, local services and referral pathways.

OOH care has also changed over the past few decades. Initially, general practice principals were contractually obliged to provide round-the-clock cover for their own patients. In the 1990s co-operatives began to emerge where practices would join together to provide out-of-hours care, but it remained the responsibility of the practices themselves to ensure that good medical cover was in place. Since the 2004 contract, the Primary Care Organ-isation (PCO) has the responsibility to deliver OOH services, and they may commission private companies or co-operatives of local surgeries working together. As for locum cover, it remains the responsibility of the GP Princi-pal and their team to ensure suitable cover in their absence, or – in the case of a (PCO) run practice – the responsibility of the PCO.

Pros and cons

Inherent in both modes of working is flexibility, giving choice of where, when and for whom one works. This career pattern can allow maintenance of a good life-work balance. For some, it means the ability to pursue an alternative career, either medical or non-medical, whilst keeping one's skills up-to-date. Within the medical sphere, it is possible to pursue academic, political, or other interests. Local Medical Committees (LMCs are groups of General Practitioners who represent the profession, and negotiate on issues facing primary care) and the Royal College of General Practitioners are increasingly seeking the input of sessional GPs on issues such as revalida-tion. Shorter-term commitments enable you to take time away, for instance, on expeditions as discussed in Chapter 9: International primary care, or for other sabbatical positions. Equally it might allow you time to pursue non-medical interests, such as painting, sailing or spending more time with your family.

However, there are also disadvantages. With both locum and OOH work, there is less security and stability. The amount of available work can fluctuate, so at times whatever work is offered has to be taken, and it can be hard to safeguard your own need for blocks of time away for annual leave, or attending courses. At other times, you will be turning down offers of work. This is more often the case during school and public holidays. A locum may also be required to cover sick leave, maternity leave, or to work in challenging areas where there are recruitment difficulties.

Both locum and OOH work can be an excellent means of getting to grips with the variety of settings in which primary care can be delivered. This 'bird's eye view' gives you a unique breadth of experience, working with different teams, population groups and systems. It can be a way of understanding and developing your own professional identity – what is important to you in the way that you practise your art. It allows you to earn a living, whilst clarifying the type of work you may wish to commit to. Also, the breadth of local knowledge can make you a valuable contributor on local issues for the LMC or PCO.

An important question for locum and OOH doctors is currently how to gather evidence of experience to use for revalidation. Specific areas which require careful consideration include gathering data towards audit and 360 degree feedback, which involves requesting comments from colleagues and patients about your day-to-day work.

Being a locum

Working as a locum provides a helpful insight into the ethos of individual practices – the atmosphere, appointment system, computer system, in-house services, working styles, and patient demographics. You can choose how much to work and tailor this to your interests, needs and financial requirements.

Such shorter-term work often means that you are less familiar with the patients, and each day can be very different. Some patients may prefer the familiarity of their usual GP, whereas others may positively value a fresh perspective. Generally, however, when working on a shorter-term basis, the focus of consultations tends toward the medical model of diagnosis and treatment and away from the more relationship-based aspects of primary care. This can be liberating, interesting and challenging. However, at times, you may miss the continuity which comes with an established relationship between patients and regular staff. Establishing rapport, working out reasons for attendance, understanding the patient's perspective, picking up cues and reaching a shared understanding may be harder to establish on a first encounter. Thus, the importance of good communication cannot be overemphasised, both in establishing the most satisfying consultations for doctor and patient, and in avoiding complaints.

Although it is difficult to get exact figures, the Medical Protection Society (MPS) suggest there are possibly a higher proportion of complaints against locum doctors than against Salaried and Principal GPs. This may be partly because it is easier to complain against a relatively unfamiliar doctor than the one with whom the patient has on-going ties. This means that you need to be especially thorough as a locum, despite being in unfamiliar surroundings. According to the MPS, the four areas which most often cause complaints and medico-legal problems for locum GPs are consent, confidentiality, record-keeping and communication. A positive feature of being a locum is that you can leave work with fewer loose ends regarding administrative or managerial issues. The flip side of this is that you may not see the outcomes of your work.

Though it may require extra initiative, this can be addressed by active follow-up and audit of your work. Practices vary in their attitudes towards locums. At the worst end of the scale, in some practices, you may feel you are perceived as a necessary evil, with a sense of erosion of your professional autonomy within a practice that has a very idiosyncratic way of operating. At times it can be isolating, but in others, you are made to feel like a valuable and enduring member of the team, and long-term working relationships can be a very helpful source of two-way support. You can also safeguard against feeling isolated by joining a learning set, or other local medical organisation.

Keeping up-to-date with changes in service implementation and clinical developments is each doctor's own responsibility. This can be harder without access to practice meetings and the informal discussions that team members often share.

It can seem foreign at the outset to negotiate fees for yourself, but this may also add to your repertoire of skills. The paperwork involved in locum work is not onerous, but requires a certain level of organisation to keep a running record of work done, invoices sent, payment received, as well as pension and tax payments made.

OOH work

Sometimes patients feel confused about the exact role of the OOH GP service, therefore, a part of OOH consultations is the management of patient expectations. With such political emphasis on access and choice, it is hardly surprising that this confusion exists. Often, patients assume that the OOH team has full access to patient records. At present, however, OOH care often relies on a verbal account from the patient of their relevant medical history and list of medications, although some additional information may be available via the patient Summary Care Record (SCR).

There are many ways to access OOH care and the amount of triage performed will have an impact upon the type of problems you deal with. It is not uncommon for patients to present seeking reassurance or information about management of more medically minor conditions such as coughs, colds and gastroenteritis, particularly for patients at either age extreme. OOH services also commonly support patients who are feeling unable to cope at home in some way, for example the elderly (perhaps lonely and suffering from multiple chronic illnesses), or patients with an exacerbation of a mental illness (such as worsening depression or anxiety, addiction or psychosis). Supporting these patients and their families in the short-term, while also defining the best long-term strategies and follow-up with their usual day-time professional teams, can prove both rewarding and challenging.

It can be interesting to work in a way that is different to the normal general practice day. During OOH shifts, you may use more telephone communication skills and apply a more medical model of dealing with presentations. Working solely in OOH care, there may be a danger of de-skilling in the management of chronic disease, such as diabetic care and wider health surveillance. On the other hand, the skills developed in managing acute problems effectively in OOH are readily transferable to other GP settings.

Generally, there is a high demand for doctors to cover OOH shifts, and so it is relatively easy to get involved in this type of work. It is an interesting way to understand your local primary care provision and to meet local colleagues. In the OOH service, there may well be time-targets which you are encouraged to help meet (clinical need permitting), but there is rarely a well-defined appointment system. This can result in lulls or 'pile ups'. On the other hand, the lack of fixed appointment times can allow you to explore the presenting problem with the patient in a more satisfying way, without the sense of overrunning.

Medical Defence Union (MDU) review shows that although 70% of the week is covered by OOH care, only 8% of all complaints in primary care received by them in 2005 and 2006 arose from OOH care (Green, 2007). In almost all complaints communication issues were involved, even if this was not the primary cause of complaint.

Practical advice

How to get work

There are a number of ways to get yourself known in the local area, for example, attending education sessions, and contacting your local PCO who will often assimilate an email list of locums to whom they will cascade available sessions. You can also approach practices directly and your local deanery will keep a list of teaching practices. A simple letter or email introducing yourself, your qualifications and availability may suffice. You will tend to have a higher response rate if you enclose a Curriculum Vitae (CV) as this gives a fuller picture of you as a practising doctor. As you become established, working relationships with particular practices may develop and the 'grapevine' will often bring further work. Practices with which you have established a relationship can be helpful in recommending you to others.

Alternatively you can join a local 'chambers' if there is one. This can be a great way of further professionalising your role, fostering a sense of belonging, gaining administrative and practical support, having a voice in the local area and participating in educational and personal development. A chambers can provide a more robust framework within which to address revalidation.

The many locum agencies vary in their quality. So prior to signing up to a particular contract, it is worth asking what sort of work they commonly have available. Many of these agencies have a relatively specific geographic or service area (e.g. military posts). One advantage is that they often organise and pay for your Criminal Record Bureau (CRB) check. Take time to read the contracts in advance to clarify whether taking work through them will prevent you working with the same practices in future through independent contracts. Currently, any salary through a locum agency is not superannuable, i.e., does not count towards contributions to the NHS Pension scheme.

Regarding OOH work, there are a number of providers who cover different parts of the UK. Simply ask colleagues locally to find out whom to approach. You may be required to register and attend an induction. Once on their books, you should be able to sign up for their sessions.

Negotiating

Even at times when there appears to be a surplus of locum doctors in your area, practices will almost always still be struggling with a lack of 'good locums'. You can establish a good reputation by being reliable, courteous, communicative and providing good clinical care. It is important to be clear about mutual expectations.

Local rates of pay can be found out from local colleagues or your local National Association for Sessional General Practitioners (NASGP) representative and are regularly published in the trade magazines *Pulse* or *GP*. You can negotiate with each practice for either a sessional or an hourly rate. Also negotiable is the number of patients you see, whether you will do home visits, or repeat prescriptions, and how long you would like for your appointments. Working as a locum does involve adjusting to a new environment, so it is justifiable to ask for longer consultations or some catch-up time. It is important to negotiate a pattern of working that supports you in providing good, safe clinical care to all the patients you see. Remember when negotiating fees that your income accounts for annual, study and sick leave. There is helpful guidance for negotiating fees for locum GPs on the BMA website (www.bma.org).

OOH providers usually have a fixed rate of pay, with rates varying depending on the shift length and whether it is a weekend, night, or bank holiday. Be sure to clarify whether the OOH provided pays pension contributions. Unlike locum work, there is usually little room for negotiation.

Paperwork

You will need to provide original documentation of:
➤ General Medical Council membership
➤ Certificate of Completion of Training or MRCGP
➤ Professional Indemnity with either Medical Defence Union (MDU) or Medical Protection Society (MPS)
➤ Criminal Records Bureau (CRB) status
➤ Hepatitis B status
➤ Primary Care Organisation (PCO) Performer's List
➤ Qualifications (Medical Degree, postgraduate qualifications).

You might like to have these documents as a pdf file, so that it is easy to send to practices when required. It can be important to keep written contracts between yourself and the practice detailing dates, times, any additional duties and rates of pay agreed. The NASGP has models for these, but an email will suffice as a paper agreement.

Induction

Ideally, when you arrive to begin locum work for the first time in a practice or OOH setting, you will be taken through an induction which should include an introduction to the computer system. Having your own personal log-on is a medico-legal requirement and a way of assimilating data for audit. It can be helpful, if you are a member of the NASGP, to take a look at their online pages introducing you to a number of different computer software packages in use. Often, you will be provided with an information pack of internal and external contact information. It can be very useful to have a person in-house whom you can contact with questions; referral pathways; where things are; protocols; and ideally a box with some equipment available so that you do not have to spend valuable time hunting through drawers for prescription pads, medical certificates, peak flow meters, blood forms, sample pots etc.

Again, the NASGP has prepared a suggested template for Practice Induction Packs and this may be worth suggesting to practices if necessary.

Handover

Perhaps there is a test result which must not be overlooked, or you want to ensure that a certain patient books a follow-up appointment in a fortnight. Make sure that you are familiar with practice handover procedures and know which GP to handover to (and if they are about to go on annual leave, their deputy!). You are likely to manage anxiety about patients in a different way as a locum, as you cannot be reassured by follow-up through investigations and a second consultation in the same way as a regular GP. You must, therefore, be aware of any existing practice procedures and know how to use these not only to ensure good clinical care for your patients but also to satisfy your own professional expectations.

Finance

Some locums will take an invoice with them on the day, whilst others will send off invoices in a batch at the end of the month. It is simple enough to develop a spreadsheet of work done, when pay has been received, and how much to set aside for tax and pension. It is important to keep business records, retaining copies of invoices and pension records.

You will need to register immediately with HM Revenue and Customs as self-employed in order to avoid paying a penalty, and to start paying Class 2 and 4 National Insurance contributions.

It can be invaluable to employ an accountant who will calculate your income tax and complete your self-assessment tax forms, potentially saving you money.

You will need to check whether the work you do is superannuable. Work in GMS, PMS or APMS surgeries will be superannuable, but OOH work may not be (*see* Chapter 2 on salaried jobs and partnerships for a fuller explanation of the different sorts of practices). The NHS pensions website gives more information, and the specific documents can be found in the section 'members forms' where GP locum forms A and B are filed. You must complete a locum form A for each separate employer in the month, and one locum form B, which summarises all sources of pensionable pay during the month. These are then returned to the pension officer of your PCO within ten weeks of the completion of work.

Organisations

Make sure that you are paying enough Medico-legal defence cover for the number of sessions you undertake. As locum doctors do not necessarily have a regular workload, the defence organisations will be able to tell you how many sessions you are covered for annually, as well as weekly. The Medical Protection Society has a publication 'Sessional GP' freely accessible online with much helpful information and advice.

Being an independent practitioner makes it even more important to have the support of the BMA in case of any disputes or difficulties. The NASGP is also an excellent source of practical support and cross-fertilisation of ideas and networks. They will also send you an up-to-date copy of the British National Formulary (BNF) bi-annually, if you prefer a paper version (www. bnf.org).

Education

It is a good idea to try to attend practice meetings, even if you do not receive payment for this time, as it gives you the opportunity to keep abreast of debates within the medical landscape.

The responsibility rests solely on the shoulders of the locum or OOH doctor to keep themselves and any relevant documentation up-to-date. Joining or establishing a learning group is also a good way to meet colleagues and manage your on-going development, as well as building a network for support and advice. The local postgraduate education centre will also regularly run primary care teaching.

Without the continuity of care inherent in regular posts, it can be difficult to keep track of your performance. Do your best to obtain meaningful feedback, which will form a part of your appraisal and help you to establish your professional development plan (PDP). There are useful feedback forms prepared by the NASGP.

There are now plenty of online learning resources through BMJ learning (free to BMA members), doctors.net, and e-learning for health, as well as the RCGP online modules which are ideal for flexible education and for providing 'evidence' of what you have done.

Personal development

Whereas some salaried GPs have time built into their contract for personal development, locum and OOH doctors do not. Some Deaneries offer mentoring schemes, often for GPs who have recently finished training schemes. These can be a great source of help in formulating your ideas about career progression and support for your well-being.

Appraisal

Usually appraisals are the responsibility of the PCO with whom you are registered on a Performer's List. Despite the importance of participation, both as a helpful means of personal learning and reflection, and as the regulatory cornerstone of the revalidation process, low uptake of appraisals by locum GPs has been a concern in some parts of the UK.

With the introduction of a new system of complaints in April 2009, by the Department of Health, a practice is now required to contact you directly for a fact-finding interview or witness statement should a complaint be made against you. It is worth checking with your PCO how many sessions you need to do in their area in order to qualify for payment towards appraisal completion and preparation.

Given the often disperse and sporadic nature of locum and OOH work, it is worth trying to build in time for regular reflection and completion of learning tasks for your appraisal during your working week (www.appraisals.nhs.uk). For more information on professional development, *see* Chapter 7.

Revalidation

The streamlining of the revalidation and relicensing process by the GMC and RCGP is evolving but remains focussed around the appraisal process. The GMC website has a downloadable working framework for appraisal and assessment which can stimulate thought on how to provide more summative elements of evidence to meet the criteria.

Summary

Doctors working as locums and in Out-of-Hours services represent a significant proportion of the primary care workforce. This style of working is inherently flexible, but can also be less stable. The challenges are slightly different to those faced by General Practitioners in a regular post, and tend to be centred round adapting to new environments and people. Often the consultations in these contexts tend to become more about medical, rather than psychosocial aspects of patient care, but not always.

There are many advantages to being able to manage your own timetable and to having the variety this offers. It is a style of working that some doctors thrive on, many choosing this as their permanent career.

Sources of further information

The National Association of Sessional GPs	www.nasgp.org.uk
The NHS Pensions Agency	www.nhsbsa.nhs.uk
HM Revenue and Customs	www.hmrc.gov.uk
General Medical Council	www.gmc-uk.org
Medical Defence Union	www.the-mdu.com
Medical Protection Society	www.medicalprotection.org/uk
The NHS Spine	www.connectingforhealth.nhs.uk
BMA	www.bma.org.uk

Reference

Green S. *A Review of Out of Hours Complaints and Claims in Primary Care* London: Medical Defence Union, 2007.

Career profile:

Sarah Donald

When did you qualify?
BSc Hons Nutrition 1997
MBChB 2002
MRCGP 2007

What is your job?
I now work permanently as a salaried GP part-time in a rural practice where I have a special interest in Diabetes. I also have a regular commitment to providing out-of-hours care in the far remote North West of Scotland and locum for other practices in the area.

Why and how did you choose general practice?
I chose general practice because of the variety of work, the ability to pursue specialty work (the portfolio career) and the lifestyle.

Where did you work?
I trained in Edinburgh and the Scottish Borders. I then travelled to Australia and New Zealand where I worked in Sydney and Christchurch in A&E posts before returning to the Scottish Highlands to complete my GP training. Once qualified with my MRCGP, I did a further year training as a Remote and Rural Fellow in the North of Scotland. This gave me the opportunity to work across a number of practices of varying sizes and remoteness. Some were single-handed small practices while other practices were larger with community hospital commitments. I also had the time and options to set my own learning needs to become a more rounded rural GP and spent some time gaining Family Planning and Minor Surgical skills as well as familiarity with dispensing and practice management styles.

What is the most rewarding aspect of your job?
I love having the ability to choose when and where I work but also having the continuity of knowing the area and its community.

What is the most challenging or frustrating thing about your job?
Working across an extensive geographical area is both a challenge but enormously rewarding. The multidisciplinary team within the area have developed excellent communication skills and members frequently extend their roles beyond that which they are employed.

If you could change one thing about your career, what would it be?

Nothing!

What do you wish you knew then that you know now?

Do not listen to colleagues who tell you that a stint working abroad will damage your career prospects. Everyone I know who has spent some time travelling and working abroad has done exceptionally well in whichever career path they have chosen and are probably a more balanced person as a result.

Reflective piece: 'Out-of-hours work'

Sophie Kuhn

I am trying to tie together loose ends from a recent afternoon surgery before heading out the door; it is always a mad dash to reach the out-of-hours service on time. It is never convenient to work in the evening or at weekends as it is a sacrifice of time that could be spent with family or friends. But there are more rewards to working out-of-hours than purely financial ones.

There is a degree of anticipation in finding out who the driver (with whom I will be spending the next six hours) will be. Being driven in a warm car, listening to the football or 'Magic' radio can be soporific. On arrival at the patient's home I give my arm a pinch to remind myself that I am still a doctor on duty, as I have perfected the art of leaving my work and role behind at the end of a day.

For those with a curiosity about how other people live it is a great privilege to visit patients in their own home. We go from extreme affluence to extreme poverty, from one culture to another. In addition to the details provided by a patient, there is a wealth of information to be gained from just looking around the living room. A shift in power occurs from doctor to patient. I have often wondered why it takes so much longer to see a patient at home than in surgery. One of the reasons is that in the home setting, the patient invariably takes the opportunity to divert the conversation away from his medical problems. To avoid this I make a conscious effort to sit as though in a surgery, turn off the television and ask relatives to leave unless they are carers or translators.

The preamble to a call written by a triaging doctor at one of the bases can really be of help if read properly! I learnt this from bitter experience when I once skimmed though a call sheet, noting only the word 'diabetic'. As I approached the house the door was wide open. When I tried to shut the door a police officer startled me, while I was even more shocked when I entered the bedroom to come across a gory battle scene that had come to a sad end. A thin old man lay, motionless, white as a sheet and covered in dried blood, dead. Was this the scene of a murder? Thoughts were flashing through my mind as a second officer approached to question me. I looked down nervously at my call sheet and realised that my visit was meant to be a simple confirmation of death. It is amazing how, if caught off guard, human emotions, which have been otherwise desensitised through repeated exposure to death, kick in.

It is a privilege to have a driver who finds the address and accompanies you in dangerous areas. A medical bag is a tempting target. Moreover, in the home I am invariably overwhelmed by the respect and gratitude shown.

It is especially rewarding to visit the elderly and house-bound patients at home. It may just be a simple infection, pain control or reassurance which can easily be dealt with at home using the medication we carry, thus avoiding the upheaval and expense of a hospital admission.

Every case is self-contained with no follow-up and there is little stress as you can only go as fast as the car will take you to the next house call. It also feels much lighter in terms of responsibility compared to my surgery as one either treats the patient, refers him to the hospital or his GP if follow-up is required for complex social problems and long-term conditions. This may be you the next day.

CHAPTER 5

GPs with a special interest

Dominic Roberts and Sophie Park

Such doctors must be good GPs first and foremost and they must deliver their special interest within their generalist care. We do not wish to see a fragmentation of general practice with the devaluing and eventual loss of generalism to the detriment of patient care as occurred to the general physician.

Dobson, 2001

The notion of a 'specialist' within general practice (GPwSI) may seem like a contradiction. This chapter will attempt to clarify the potentially blurred professional boundaries between 'generalism' and 'specialism' and also show how these roles are highly influenced by the wider political changes in the NHS. Much of this chapter is informed by the experience of a GP principal with a special interest in Ear Nose and Throat (ENT). This is particularly relevant, as the route to developing a specialist interest role is currently quite ad hoc, reflecting doctors' own circumstances or interests, as well as the service requirements in a given area. Nevertheless, we hope this chapter will be useful to you, either helping you to understand as a GP where GPwSIs fit into the broader landscape, or conveying some guiding principles that will help you think about whether becoming a GPwSI is the right career move for you. You will also find some practical tips for getting a specialist service up and running.

Origins of the GPwSI

In defining what a GPwSI is or does, it may be useful to briefly consider the role of a 'normal GP'. What is a specialist and what is a generalist? General practice has become recognised as a specialty in itself over a number of years. This reflects the unique context in which doctors are seeing patients, the needs they address and as Roger Neighbour explains in his Foreword the lens they use in defining and approaching problems. They have become expert not only in the management of many chronic conditions such as diabetes, depression and cardiovascular disease but also in balancing the treatment of patients who have multiple pathologies. Many GPs within a practice take on responsibility for co-ordinating and updating the practice in a particular clinical field and, as such, may develop specialist knowledge within the spectrum of the General Practitioner role, which they share with their practice team. These 'specialisms' may reflect clinical experience prior to training in general practice, or represent specialist knowledge learned during the job in order to address the needs of a particular patient population, such as drug or alcohol misuse.

Essentially, becoming a GPwSI is an extension of this specialism. Being a GPwSI implies you have specialist knowledge which goes *beyond* that of most GPs. Some may argue that the concept of a GPwSI is something that has existed in general practice for many years; 'GPwSI' being merely a new title for practitioners who have had a special interest or clinical experience in a particular field for a long time. Historically, GPs who had a particular extensive interest in, for example, Dermatology or Paediatrics might have worked as 'associate specialists' in hospital clinics, but also shared their knowledge with their primary care colleagues and provided a second opinion.

There has then been some contention about what exactly makes someone a GPwSI and at what stage someone can adopt that label. Does simply having a special interest convey this title? Who decides whether you can adopt the title? What regulation exists to ensure you are keeping up-to-date and practicing safely and effectively? These are questions for which consensus is slowly being reached, with historical parallels to the 19th century debates regarding who could adopt the official label of 'doctor.'

More recently, accreditation has been formalised and resulted in a more explicit definition of a GPwSI. For instance, it is now a Department of Health (DoH) requirement that all practising GPwSIs are formally accredited by their Primary Care Organisation (PCO), the requisites of which are detailed later in this chapter. This has been largely welcomed by GPwSI professionals, defining more formal boundaries and regulation surrounding who can call themselves a GPwSI. The Association of Practitioners with a Special Interest (www.apwsi.co.uk) is a national organisation offering professional support to those who practice as a GPwSI and publish a regular journal. Formally identifying and offering a title of GPwSI offers huge benefits in recognising their contribution, enabling regulation and allowing their talents to be maximised by local primary care networks. Proponents of this formalisation hoped that this would result in decreased referral rates as well and offer added value for the taxpayer.

The Rationale

The traditional model of care in general practice involves most patients being assessed and treated by the GP themselves. Some patients may, however, be referred to a specialist to address a patient's needs. For example, a referral may be useful in allowing a patient to accept their illness, or prognosis; a GP may recognise that the management plan required exceeds their own knowledge; or the patient requires a specialist procedure or facilities. GPwSIs represent an augmentation of this system. For example, if a patient has a sebaceous cyst and there is a GP who runs a clinic in minor surgery down the road, then it might be far more convenient, just as safe and more cost effective to refer the patient there, rather than to a hospital with longer waiting lists which may be some distance away.

Discussions about cost effectiveness and competing providers of similar services have become far more common in general practice with the increasing role of quasi-markets in the NHS (DOH 2010; Pollock, 2004). Within the White Paper 'Liberating the NHS', GPs have been allocated a significant role in practice-based commissioning (PBC) – the process by which GPs procure appropriate services for their patients, usually with different providers (NHS or private companies) bidding for the contract. This produces some new challenges within the doctor-patient relationship as GPs explore the explicit tensions within their role responsibilities, including both patient advocate and rationing resources.

There has been much debate about GPwSIs in the literature, particularly by making cost comparisons with consultant consultations and patient satisfaction. There are still some unanswered questions as to whether GPwSIs genuinely offer value for money compared to secondary care services. One randomised controlled trial comparing a GPwSI-led service for skin disease and a hospital dermatology service found favourable outcomes towards the GPwSI clinic on parameters such as accessibility and patient satisfaction. Furthermore, no noticeable difference was found in clinical outcomes between the two services (Salisbury 2005).

Some studies suggest that GPwSI services are significantly more costly to the health service than secondary care for broadly similar clinical outcomes, with caveats that the financial costs be balanced against the benefits of advanced access for patients (Coast, 2005). Other GPwSI services have demonstrated that they are considerably more cost effective than secondary care, for example in dermatology, consultations costing £23:35 versus five times this cost for consultant care (Crowley, 2006). Similarly, a GPwSI-led headache service in London had higher patient satisfaction rates and similar outcomes, but for lower cost than their secondary care counterpart (Ridsdale, 2008). In summary, analyses appear to show wide variation in the cost of services being run throughout the country, partly also dependent upon which measures (such as money versus patient satisfaction) are most valued within the research analysis.

Why become a GPwSI rather than a Consultant?

The two are very different. The striking difference is that a GPwSI is not a specialty or job in its own right, but an extended role that compliments that of a general practitioner. Most GPwSIs perform their role part-time with general practice being their main profession. This might, therefore, bring the benefits of having a special interest yet also being able to enjoy the full benefits of general practice; patient continuity; clinical variety; community care; independence and flexible working. Being a consultant obviously has its own merits and, if being a specialist is something which attracts you most, you may be more suited to this profession.

You may be at the stage where you are deciding whether to pursue a career as a hospital specialist or GP. Being a GPwSI provides some compromise to an extent, giving you an area of subject expertise whilst facilitating a dual role as a generalist. These roles may, however, contrast considerably.

A significant proportion of patients in general practice have no specific 'medicalised' diagnosis and require support from their GPs for a myriad of diverse and complex problems, often utilising their relationship with the GP as well as more practical help to maximise their function. This requires different consultation skills to those focussed upon in hospital, using patients' own notions of health and illness, concerns, expectations and time, in addition to making numerous judgements differentiating between possible diagnoses and a range of suitable investigations and trials of treatment (Stewart, 2001). This tolerance of uncertainty may be very different in specialist clinics. There, patients have already been through a selection process, refined their stories and have a provisional diagnosis made, warranting further (often more invasive) investigation.

These different approaches and levels of certainty may appeal to different people. Providing a committed service to patients in general practice can be highly rewarding, but can also be exhausting and draining. There are many ways to address this. Choosing to cultivate an interest in a particular area may be one way to achieve a rewarding addition to the working week, providing a variety of stimuli and exposing you to differing patient needs. This change may be refreshing for some and in fact improve your performance within general practice, as well as offering personal opportunities for professional development.

Why become a GPwSI and not a Generalist? By definition of a GPwSI, it is not possible for you to become a GPwSI without, first and foremost, being a GP. Technically it might be possible to spend most of your time as a GPwSI, rather than a GP, but this would be unusual. Being a GPwSI is not a specialty in its own right, but more an extension of one's role as a GP, the advantages of which are outlined below.

Benefits of being a GPwSI

There are many benefits to being a GPwSI:

➤ It enables you to pursue a special clinical interest. One of the negative perceptions of general practice, as Roger Neighbour highlights in his Foreword, is the concept that you are a 'jack of all trades but a master of none'. In reality, the depth and breadth of a GP's knowledge tends to be constantly shaped and adapted to meet the needs of their patients. While it is important to recognise when something feels 'out of your depth', this can just as often reflect patient-orientated and personality challenges, as limitations in knowledge fields. However, despite the variety and challenge of general practice surgeries, some GPs may wish at some point to develop an additional element to vary their working week. Being a GPwSI allows you to focus and develop a particular clinical flare and can facilitate an increase in confidence, managing patients within your general practice with problems related to your special interest.

➤ The working environment, particularly if working within a hospital setting with consultants, hospital colleagues and networking with other GPwSIs, can be quite different, focussing on team, rather than individual responsibility for a patient's care. Developing new professional relationships can enrich both your own and colleagues' practice. For example, conversations in clinic or regularly attending dermatology conferences can provide an opportunity to network and discuss ideas informing your patient care.

➤ Working as a GPwSI can offer personal satisfaction in feeling competent within a particular field. GPs become expert in managing uncertainty which exists within daily practice, defining boundaries of knowledge (in keeping personally up-to-date and accepting the limits of current evidence for a specific situation); patient circumstances and relationships; rationing; recognising levels of confidence and acting appropriately (Beresford, 1991). Developing a special interest in a particular field, in addition to close liaison with hospital specialists can bring the opportunity to focus on a particular subject area with an increase in certainty, which some clinicians enjoy.

➤ The role bridges the gap between primary and secondary care, which has historically been segregated.

➤ Income varies greatly between regions, PCOs and what you negotiate from the onset of the service you create. GPwSIs tend to earn an income similar to salaried GPs (approximately £6000–£8000 per session), rather than

partnership (approximately £13 000–£15 000 per session) (Hutt, 2009).
However there is wide variation and some GPwSI's services can be quite
lucrative.

➤ You can share knowledge with colleagues in the practice. Having a special
interest allows you to lead in your field and disseminate knowledge
through teaching and tutorials in your practice. It also provides the
opportunity for colleagues to gain an expert second opinion either by
calling you in during their consultation or ringing for advice, but also by
offering the patient an appointment with you (although this has to be
carefully balanced to ensure that you help develop colleagues' knowledge
base, rather than creating a dependence in your area of expertise, and that
you maintain your usual general practice as well).

➤ Lower referral rates – having a special interest may enable you to reduce
referral rates not only personally but also in your practice. This requires
particular attention to your own awareness of boundaries and capabilities,
in order to ensure appropriate patient care. There is, conversely, some
evidence that GPs may refer more frequently if they have experience in
a particular specialty, perhaps reflecting an awareness of less common
diagnoses or facilities which may be available to patients.

➤ Being a GPwSI offers an opportunity to teach colleagues, trainees, medical
students and your local consortium, or on your local GP training scheme.
This can offer many rewards beyond that of a pay cheque.

Disadvantages to being a GPwSI:

➤ Time commitments may increase while you are gaining competence,
qualifications and expertise to practice as a GPwSI. There are also
organisational demands on your time to set up a service and run it
smoothly, for example, equipment ordering, infection control procedures
and facilitating referrals and appointments. There is also another layer
of appraisal, personal development and accreditation that you must
encompass into your time schedules. This can be rather onerous.

➤ Income for GPwSIs can be lower than partnership income (*see* above).

➤ Conflict can exist with specialists over issues such as taking referrals and
patients from secondary care facilities. This could, potentially, reduce
income to hospitals and create a feeling of 'taking our work'. It is vital,
when planning and setting up a GPwSI service, that you communicate
regularly with your local department and gain the support of at least
one of the consultants, emphasising the possible benefits for consultant
services outlined below.

➤ While most consultants accept and encourage GPwSI colleagues, some are
resentful. There is certainly a body of specialists who feel that GPwSIs are
a misnomer and that patients should see their GP and either be managed

in primary care or referred to a 'real' specialist. GPwSIs have, therefore, to constantly prove their worth by means of audit both ensuring not only quality of care but also cost effectiveness. GPwSI services will only survive if they can consistently prove they offer value for money over secondary care.

➤ As discussed above, there is conflicting evidence about cost and value for money of GPwSI services over and above consultant care.

➤ Medico-legal issues are also important, reflecting what may happen within the consultation. One could argue that working as a GPwSI potentially conveys higher clinical risk than general practice, especially where minor procedures are being carried out. It is, however, reassuring that defence fees for GPwSI work are currently identical to routine GP sessions.

➤ Many people are attracted to the notion of becoming a GPwSI when applying to general practice training. While there are certain choices during training which will help support this role, in reality, formal specialist interests are usually developed after completing nMRCGP and the local population needs are established.

Opportunities for GPwSIs

GPs can train to become GPwSIs in a wide variety of clinical specialties such as:

➤ ENT
➤ Dermatology and minor surgery
➤ Ophthalmology
➤ Family planning
➤ Musculoskeletal medicine and sports medicine
➤ Public health
➤ Cardiology
➤ Respiratory medicine
➤ Allergies

And many more…

How to get started

Getting training and experience to become a GPwSI can be straightforward. Approach your PCO with an idea, particularly if you see a niche that has not been developed, and see if they are interested in supporting you. Many PCOs offer training in specific subjects as part of salaried schemes, allowing them to meet particular service needs. Equally, if you are thinking about setting up a service, you will need to get the support and backing of local secondary care consultants. It is extremely difficult to develop a GPwSI service without this support, so bring them 'on board' early. Ask if you can sit in on some clinics and gain expertise. Your PCO may fund your time there and you may be given the opportunity to run your own clinics with consultant support. Discuss your ideas and plans with the consultant. Most consultants will be supportive but beware of the possible conflict of interest in taking their patients and potentially their income. Be sensitive in your approach. Undertake a diploma designed for GPwSI training in your field and apply to the PCO to fund it.

Several factors are often helpful and sometimes essential to support a training opportunity in a particular subject:

➤ Your own personal desire and motivation is essential. Training may involve a transient reduction in income and extra time to do sessions. There will likely be a diploma in your chosen field which will require some degree of stamina and determination to achieve.

➤ Previous clinical experience in your specialist field is likely to be valuable and useful to emphasise when proposing to become a GPwSI.

➤ The training opportunity itself may be part of an existing scheme set up by a local PCO incorporating weekly sessions into a salaried GP post. The PCO may support the training in a field where a GPwSI is required. It is possible to arrange your own training by means of contacting a local consultant to observe or participate in specialist sessions. This could be done individually or, preferably, with the support of your practice.

➤ Consultant support is paramount as it will be required for training and setting up the GPwSI service itself. It would be very hard to flourish without this.

➤ Support from your practice is required to facilitate time out from practice commitments and possibly contribute to funding or partial funding of the training. This will depend on the benefit to the practice that your gained expertise brings, which should be relatively easy to demonstrate.

➤ PCO support may be both financial and logistical, arranging training and setting up of the service, in addition to keeping you abreast of any local discussions regarding Practice Based Commissioning (PBC).

There are potential benefits to your local consultants in setting up a service and emphasise these early. These include:

➤ Potential extra income for consultant training time, (if the PCO will fund it).

➤ It may be that you will be able to run your own clinic, alongside the consultant, during your training period and this can increase clinical capacity for the hospital. This in turn helps with access and waiting times. Your clinic will be similar in structure to that of a year two foundation doctor (FY2), in that you will have consultant or registrar support at all times.

➤ It can provide the consultant with an opportunity to get to know their local GP colleagues. GPs are often impressed that a consultant is willing to support a community service and will often invite them to give teaching about the service, common conditions and management.

➤ Similarly, it may raise the consultant's local profile. Supporting a GPwSI service will involve close liaison with you and other primary healthcare providers and will certainly improve their recognition among local GPs. This may boost support for their secondary care service, both NHS and private. This has gained particular importance since the development of the 'Choose and Book' system for referrals from primary care promoting the notion of the patient as 'consumer' with competition between recommended service providers.

➤ Your consultant will, more than likely, be involved in providing some of the clinical care in your service and will usually do a regular clinic either alongside yours or in a supervisory role to your practice. This will be remunerated and provide further income for the consultant. While it is unlikely to lead to income comparable to private practice, there is normally scope for negotiation between the consultant and provider. Most GPwSIs usually have consultant support and supervision, and this is very much encouraged.

Setting up the clinic

Realistically, you will need support from either your PCO, practice-based commissioning organisation or consortium to set up a service. Begin by out-lining a business plan – either undertaken by you, or by a manager skilled in such tasks. Your income will likely be the national tariff rates for out-patient appointments, or below to offer savings to the PCO. Outgoings will include your personal income, equipment, other staff and the appointments service. Be prepared for a long wait before your service begins as there is much red tape to overcome before you are able to start seeing patients. A service may typically take more than twelve months to get off the ground, from initial planning to seeing your first patient. For an example of a GP who developed an interest in emergency medicine see David Whittington's profile at the end of this chapter.

Professional labels

As a GPwSI, you will have expertise in your particular field, which will no doubt lead to increased confidence and ability to deal with clinical situations that previously warranted referral. It is important that you always acknowledge, both to yourself and colleagues and more importantly to patients, that you are a GP first and foremost, who has undergone some extra training in your specialty. This is vital to ensure patient trust. This difference between a GPwSI and a consultant specialist is equally important to your own decision whether to become a GPwSI. If your primary interest is to be a GPwSI rather than a GP, you may need to think again!

Know your limitations

> 'General practitioners with special interests should not practice in isolation and should have easy access to advice, support, and professional development from local hospital specialists'
>
> Rosen, 2003

As a GP with a special interest, it is important to know your clinical boundaries and when to refer to a consultant or seek advice. While you will have a broad repertoire of expertise from general practice and your experience as a GPwSI, a little specialist knowledge could cultivate over-confidence. Potentially, as a GPwSI, you may be dealing with more risky clinical situations and it is important to involve the advice and expertise of your fellow consultants when necessary. This is to avoid the risk of an adverse clinical incident and ensure on-going training and experience with consultant guidance. These professional conversations can be an invaluable source of learning to both parties. Generally speaking, patients with serious diagnoses such as cancer or suspicion of such diagnoses should be under the care of a consultant and avoiding delay is vital.

There are many specialties (listed above) who already lend themselves well to GPwSI roles. There is unlikely to be any clinical specialty that would not facilitate a role as a GPwSI in some form. In surgical specialties, there is a limit to the extent of involvement a GPwSI should safely have, with minor procedures being commonplace. An ENT GPwSI, for example, might perform laryngoscopies, micro-suction, audiometry and nasal cautery for epistaxis without supervision. Tonsillectomy would certainly be a step too far. Although some procedures may be considered straightforward, the available facilities, ability and experience of a doctor in dealing with *complications* is important. Awareness of limitations in terms of training and experience is paramount.

Indemnity and accreditation

Indemnity fees are currently the same cost as for ordinary GP sessions. You should be accredited in your specialist field in accordance with Department of Health (DoH) guidance and your indemnity provider should be informed. Given your primary role as GP, the issues surrounding risk management within the consultation are likely to be similar. As discussed above, some GPs with experience in a particular specialty are **more** likely to refer, potentially, however, a GPwSI practising in general practice may be less likely to refer patients within their specialty field, requiring constant and careful reflection within each consultation upon appropriate boundaries and confidence.

You must be accredited in accordance with the DoH guidance and this should be arranged through your PCO. Normally, a panel incorporating a consultant from another area is used to assess your portfolio, which should outline your experience and evidence and how your service works. There is a long and detailed standard application form on the DoH website which you can download (www.dh.gov.uk/publications). Ensure your PCO is aware of your service, particularly if you are seeing patients referred by other practices. Your local infection control team should inspect your premises to ensure health and safety.

Once you have undergone the necessary training and qualifications to become a GPwSI, you will need to keep up-to-date. This should normally be done by working or liaising closely with your local consultant counterpart. This is vital. Some evidence suggests that a few GPwSIs are not participating in the nationally agreed level of on-going training (Schofield, 2005). This does, of course, depend upon how learning is defined. Most of your learning will probably result from seeing patients, but as with all specialties now, you will need to keep a careful portfolio to demonstrate this learning.

The future

Politics and its impact on the provision of healthcare are ever-changing. Even if the GPWSI label is not retained the concept of a GP with a special interest is more than likely to exist within healthcare provision in some form or other. If your service addresses patients' needs well, and can be proven to be cost effective and provide value for money, in comparison to your counterpart secondary care service, you are likely to stay afloat.

It is, however, worth carefully considering your career choice *before* embarking upon lengthy training and planning. Although, as with many careers, the job may change by the time you have completed the training, the principles of a generalist or specialist approach to practice are unlikely to alter hugely. It is, therefore, perhaps helpful to reiterate that you should ask yourself whether you wish to be a General Practitioner or a Consultant Specialist, not whether you want to be a Consultant or a GPwSI. Being a GPwSI is an adjunct to general practice, not a career in its own right. While you will still see patients either way, the approach you use, environment in which you work and external constraints upon your practice, may differ widely.

Conclusion

Being a GPwSI potentially offers huge benefits to your career and is likely to enrich your experience in primary care in many different ways. While there are some constraints and extra time commitments involved, these are generally far outweighed by the opportunities and experience you gain, *if* it is the right career for you. The hurdles you will have to overcome to become trained and accredited should eventually enhance your professional practice. Setting up a GPwSI service from scratch can be both time consuming and at times frustrating, but will likely be overshadowed by excitement when your first patient walks into your clinic.

General practice and the provision of primary care services are changing. There are challenges ahead for GPwSIs, establishing their role within an evolving NHS, and there is a continued responsibility to ensure provision of an effective and safe service amidst a politically uncertain future. There are, however, many opportunities and potential benefits for the professional development of individual GPwSI doctors and the practices involved. Ultimately however, your role as a GPwSI, as with all GPs, is dependent upon the trust of patients (Moffat, 2006), and providing clinically effective medical care. Good Luck!

References

Beresford EB. Uncertainty and the shaping of medical decisions. *The Hastings Center Report*. 1991; **21**(4): 6–11.

Coast J, Noble S, Noble A, *et al*. Economic evaluation of a general practitioner with special interests led dermatology service in primary care. *BMJ*. 2005; **331**: 1444–1449.

Crowley C. Are GPs who specialise in dermatology effective? High cost of general practitioners with special interests is a fallacy. *BMJ*. 2006; **332**: 54.

Dobson R. Specialist GPs must not undermine the value of generalism. *BMJ*. 2001; **322**: 1270.

DOH. *Equity and Excellence: liberating the NHS*. London: Department of Health; 2010.

Hutt P. What has happened to general practice? *BMJ Careers.* 2009; 338.

Moffat MA, Sheikh A, Price D, *et al.* Can a GP be a generalist and a specialist? Stakeholders views on a respiratory general practitioner with a special interest service in the UK. *BMC Health Services Research.* 2006; **30**(6): 62.

Pollock AM. *NHS Plc: The privatisation of our health care.* London: Verso; 2004.

Ridsdale L, Doherty J, McCrone P, *et al.* A new GP with special interest service: observational study. *Brit J Gen Pract.* 2008; **58:** 478–483.

Rosen R, Stevens R, Jones R. General practitioners with special clinical interests. *BMJ.* 2003; **327:** 460–462.

Salisbury C, Noble A, Horrocks S, *et al.* Evaluation of a general practitioner with special interest service for dermatology: randomised controlled trial. *BMJ.* 2005; **331:** 1441–1446.

Schofield JK, Irvine A, Jackson S, *et al.* General practitioners with a special interest in dermatology: results of an audit against Department of Health (DH) guidance. *Br J Derm.* 2005; **153**(1): 0–1.

Stewart M. Towards a global definition of patient centred care. *BMJ.* 2001; **322**(7284): 444–445.

Career profile:

David Whittington

When did you qualify?

I finished medical school in 1983, and completed MRCGP in 1998 after doing a self-assembled scheme, which was common in those days. Along the way I did my diplomas. I have the following qualifications; MBChD, DRCOG, DCH, MRCGP.

What is your job?

I work as a GP Principle at the Mission Practice in Bethnal Green, East London, for four sessions a week, and as a GP Consultant in Emergency Medicine at the Royal London Hospital for three sessions a week. This includes work with the Helicopter Emergency Services (HEMS). I'm also the clinical lead for one of the GP networks in our PCO, and I'm also leading on the GP care for the 2012 Olympics.

Why and how did you choose General Practice?

I made a firm commitment to inner city general practice during my second year at medical school. This was partly for religious reasons, and I eventually chose to work at a Christian Practice – which serves a diverse multicultural community in the East End. I think many patients appreciate that we have a faith, even if it differs from their own. I'm very open about my faith.

My role as a GP Emergency consultant was created for me. I don't think that there are any equivalent posts and it exists thanks to the support of the consultants at the Royal London Hospital. I guess my role is like that of a GPwSI, it arose after having done GP sessions in A&E, and had a lot do with good rapport with the PCO and consultants in the department. I'm employed on similar terms to a salaried GP.

What is the most rewarding aspect of your job?

I love the clinical independence and control that comes with the job – it's such a pragmatic specialty. As a GP, the more you see, the more rewarding it becomes. It's surprising how easy it is to keep up-to-date simply by seeing patients, reading clinic letters etc. It's also a privilege to work with mutually supportive colleagues.

What's the most challenging and frustrating thing about your job?

I think it has to be the hours. It's really hard to get the balance right between work and outside life. To provide excellent clinical care in an inner city context takes time. I realised that I wasn't able do nine sessions of face-to-face general practice; there wasn't enough time to maintain the high standards required. Apart from family and church, I don't really have much time for a social life.

If you could change one thing about your career, what would it be?

I wish I lived five minutes from my practice. We moved, mainly for school reasons, and now it takes me about an hour to travel to work.

What do you wish you knew then that you know now?

I wish I'd known how good GPs really are earlier in my career. It took me a long time to get perspective on this. I think when you work in emergency medicine you realise how important the role of the GP is. Spending part of my week in A&E, away from the often pressurised and isolated environment of the practice, has also emphasised this.

Reflective piece: 'What do you use when you have sex?

Radhika Shah

So, what do you use when you have sex?' – is not a question I am often asked by patients, but it is one that makes me smile and realise that working with young(ish) people in reproductive health, challenges all one's personal and medical boundaries.

My story of getting involved in reproductive health was initially one of disillusionment with working in a large inner city practice with high levels of deprivation. This had exposed me to a disproportionately high concentration of mental illness and physical problems that could potentially be solved if only we could write prescriptions for a suitable home and a holiday. However, working in sexual and reproductive health clinics offered me the opportunity to get involved in the provision of truly holistic and preventative healthcare to relatively healthy women and men.

One of the reasons I enjoy these clinics is that there is often no time-frame, no regularity, and no one consultation is ever the same – although one often breathes a sigh of relief in a busy reproductive health clinic if there is a 'simple pill repeat'. Yet, nothing is ever simple and there is no such thing as a typical patient either: young men wanting to know how to treat premature ejaculation; a woman in her late fifties needing counselling about an abnormal smear result, as well as a positive chlamydia test; a woman in her forties who has just given birth to twins and needs emergency contraception; and a woman in her thirties undergoing chemotherapy who needs adequate contraception. These are just a few examples of sexual and reproductive health problems that could either present to a traditional 'family planning' clinic or just as easily to the GP.

Another of the many reasons I enjoy working in this field, is that it also utilises many different skills, both practical and communicative, and there is often a great sense of teamwork in the clinics. There are opportunities to perform a wide range of procedures including: implant fittings and removals; intrauterine device (IUD) insertions; use of cryotherapy for genital warts; and ultrasound techniques for common community gynaecology problems. There are also many opportunities for training in these methods with courses and online modules. The Faculty of Sexual and Reproductive Health Diploma is very accessible using e-learning and practical sessions, and also provides study modules for more specialist areas such as menopause and vasectomy (www.ffprhc.org.uk). These are all skills that are transferable and highly beneficial in general practice. And, even if you may be unable to offer practical techniques, counselling patients about procedures is done with far more ease.

For those interested in working in the field, there are a wide variety of opportunities available; for example, in young people's drop in clinics (e.g. Brook Advisory Centres), bank doctors for local NHS clinics, clinical assistants in local hospitals and outreach clinics, and as clinical medical officers for non-governmental organisations such as the British Pregnancy Advisory Service (BPAS) and Marie Stopes. Although the pay in sexual and reproductive health is considerably lower than that of a locum GP, there are few disadvantages to working in sexual and reproductive health that come to mind. I believe that overall the genuine fulfilment of trying to provide a service of preventative and empowering healthcare is immensely satisfying.

CHAPTER 6

Academic general practice

Mareeni Raymond

The field of academic general practice has expanded hugely over the last decade and continues to receive political support for expansion. Postgraduate training has been reviewed to include more explicit career pathways and routes into academic general practice. There are expanding opportunities for both teaching and research, with a variety of ways in which to acquire training and experience.

This chapter will outline some suggestions and examples of potential routes, interests and skills, which can be developed for posts in academic general practice, as well as tips about focusing your portfolio for an academic career. Formal pathways will be discussed, as well as informal pathways for those who have already completed their training and would like to change their career to have more focus on academic practice. The wide spectrum of Academic general practice including research, educational elements or both combined will be described as well as the benefits and pitfalls of such a career. The reality of juggling clinical work, research and teaching can be challenging and, hopefully, this chapter will help to prepare you for managing these kinds of problems. It is important to remember that an academic GP can follow formal training pathways as explained in this chapter, or become involved in academic work in addition to their usual clinical duties in general practice via more informal routes to get a flavour of academic work, for example, doing research at a practice level such as audits, writing for journals and joining advisory panels. Although the focus of this chapter is on posts in undergraduate medical schools, there are many academic posts in postgraduate general practice, for example, local deaneries and the Royal College of General Practitioners (www.rcgp.org.uk). These roles are discussed in Chapter 7: Professional Development, with a focus on how to develop an interest in teaching within academia in Chapter 8: Teaching in General Practice. Finally, I will describe my experience of academic general practice, all of which will hopefully help you to make a decision about whether academic general practice is for you.

Why academia?

Academic general practice is a relatively new and exciting field, and appeals to many doctors who value the development of non-clinical skills to further enhance research and education in general practice. Academia can be deeply rewarding for those who enjoy a balance between clinical work and research activity throughout their career. In general practice there is always a need for research, particularly as primary care is constantly changing. The burden of preventive care, for example, has always been the domain of community physicians, and carrying this out on a large scale requires careful effective delivery. In recent times, the emphasis on medical management for conditions once solely the domain of secondary care has transferred to primary care, bringing a new set of responsibilities to general practitioners. This again requires research to best implement management in primary care. The scope for using research to influence and support the way doctors manage problems in primary care is huge, and the challenge appeals to many doctors.

The history of academic general practice

For years, primary care physicians have done research to enhance clinical care, albeit in a non-structured way. A clear pathway to becoming a professor of academic general practice did not exist, and depended on who knew who, who met who and who was in the right place at the right time, combined with enormous personal motivation. Recognising the need to tap into the vast data available for clinical research and the many clinicians eager to undertake this research to improve standards of clinical care and medical education, the government produced a White Paper called 'Science and Innovation: working towards a ten-year investment framework' (HM Treasury, 2004). This paper prompted the creation of the UK Clinical Research Collaboration (UKCRC) (www.ukcrc.org). Working with the NHS Modernising Medical Careers (MMC) (www.mmc.nhs.uk), guidelines for the creation of clinical academic specialty posts were produced, giving a clear idea of how a clinician could incorporate research into their career. This was in recognition of the fact that the haphazard ways that clinicians became academics were not user-friendly and that much more research could be carried out if there were a better infrastructure to do so. A joint Sub-Committee of UKCRC and MMC, Chaired by Dr Mark Walport, Director of The Wellcome Trust produced 'The Walport Report' detailing new pathways for each medical specialty (Walport, 2005).

Medical students

It is rare to know at medical student level that you want to be a GP, let alone an academic GP. However, if you have an inkling that either appeals to you, as with any other specialty, you can begin accumulating job-specific knowledge and skills particular to that field, at an early stage. This takes a lot of focussed hard work and preparation early on in your career.

The Walport Report stated that medical students should be informed about academic options and be given access to more information from their careers service. This is a good place to start, as well as by speaking to doctors already in the field of academic general practice. As with other academic specialities, the career is competitive, so the other reason to start early is to build up your CV for the challenge of gaining a post at foundation level.

Most students undertake an intercalated BSc or BA which can be very useful for learning about research and academic activity. Many students take this opportunity to try to publish their first paper by getting involved in any on-going research in their department. There even exist intercalated BScs in Primary Care at some universities such as University College London (www.ucl.ac.uk) and Leeds (www.leeds.ac.uk), which can provide excellent opportunities for primary care research at an early stage in training and an opportunity to reflect on theoretical frameworks and methods of critical analysis to apply in practice. There are hundreds of other BAs and BScs in other scientific subjects such as molecular medicine and biochemistry, but equally good are the wealth of alternative non-scientific degrees in subjects such as ethics and history of medicine. All these degrees are useful for gaining access to research opportunities and learning about different ways to approach problems. The experience may potentially influence future career paths by introducing a nugget of information that sparks an interest or a question in the student that they may later pursue in their research career. Having an intercalated degree (especially a first-class degree), prizes, published research, conference presentations and publications contributes to giving a trainee a better chance of achieving a post in academic general practice at foundation level. If a student or doctor has a desire for academic general practice, they need to constantly look for opportunities to learn, to develop new skills, and to pursue their own personal research interest with vigour as the competition for these academic posts is high.

As part of most undergraduate medical curricula, students learn about epidemiology, statistics, clinical evidence and guidelines, a good starting point to understand the principles of research. Audit opportunities in clinical years are a chance to provide evidence of some research on a CV and should be encouraged in medical school and later in clinical practice. There are two main categories of research, quantitative and qualitative, and experience in either of these will be useful to get a better understanding of the research methods used in academic practice. Quantitative research focuses on specific end points and numbers, using data that can be converted into numbers to find relationships between variables. Qualitative research requires a different set of skills to explore ideas, feelings and trends in groups of people and uses methodologies such as interviews, questionnaires, observation studies and surveys. This is so important in primary care, as the beliefs of a person can affect outcomes in diseases such as diabetes, where an understanding of diabetic control is essential to implement treatment effectively. Many academic researchers use qualitative research to collect information in the general practice setting. Some studies now combine mixed methodologies. Although you may become familiar or more comfortable with a particular epistemology or kind of knowledge (Maynard, 1994), it is probably a good idea in your early training to try and gain familiarity and experience with both approaches.

The Foundation years and Academic Foundation posts

Following medical school there are two foundation years, and getting a post in academic foundation training is competitive but useful for getting your foot in the door later on. Only certain parts of the UK offer academic posts, and to find out which universities offer them, you can look at the Society for Academic Primary Care website (www.sapc.ac.uk) or the National Institute for Health Research's Coordinating Centre for Research Capacity Development (www.nccrcd.nhs.uk).

Foundation programmes incorporating a post in academic general practice can help you decide whether the clinical side of general practice is right for you. In order to get a place on these training schemes you should ideally have evidence of research or high levels of academic attainment during medical school or in your first foundation year. Having an academic post means you are part-time in general practice and part-time in research and teaching. During that year, there is an academic theme throughout, and supervision by an academic mentor helps co-ordinate teaching, meetings, project work and research. Usually four months of the year is spent in the academic general practice post and the rest of the year consists of the typical rotations for a Foundation year.

The beauty of an academic programme is that you can work with current research projects that could impact upon general practice and usually with an influential supervisor who helps to keep track and guide your work. As an academic, you are exposed to many different professionals apart from doctors, another bonus of working in academia. This is a fantastic opportunity for you to widen the scope of ideas, share concepts and develop strategies without the bias of opinion that happens when working solely with medical doctors. These multi-professional conversations enhance reflections on clinical practice and can provide you with novel suggestions to improve approaches to practice and widen the ways that doctors think about their work.

At the beginning of your post, you should write your personal development plan, which is discussed with the supervisor before the post so that there is a clear plan for academic activity. This is vital, as without this it can be easy to get lost in the system, left doing unrelated, unimportant jobs in the department rather than working on one major project throughout and you may then leave the post with no evidence of anything significant. Unlike medical school, there are no specific objectives, notes and lecture plans. You must make the best of the opportunities for research and teaching that you come across and get the ball rolling early, as four months can pass very quickly. For MB–PhD students, there are specially designed academic foundation programmes also available.

Academic GP specialty training

After two years of foundation training, specialty training in academic general practice is an option, but it is once again competitive to gain a place. Specialty training in academic general practice is divided into an academic clinical fellowship or training phase incorporated with a higher degree, followed by a clinical lectureship phase. Some posts concentrate on research while others focus on educational training and it is up to you which path you wish to pursue. It often hard to make a decision, and tempting to continue both, but in reality, time can be very limited to do both well. You need to make sure you have a timetable, allowing enough time for every project, set goals, and get advice from a supervisor or your team regularly. Simple measures like a diary, rota and regular meetings to check on how close or far you are to your goals can make a big difference on how you cope with these various tasks.

Up to three years are spent in the clinical fellowship period, which is similar to the usual vocational training, with additional sessions kept aside in year two for academic activity. During year two, the trainee should be working with an academic department developing their own research plan for the following year while preparing their application for a training fellowship accordingly. The difficulty is in balancing clinical work with developing this research plan, and although there is time incorporated for this research, it may be that the doctor has to take their research home with them and use their spare time to work on this. During the training fellowship stage a higher degree is also obtained, such as a Masters or Doctorate in Education, or specific qualitative or quantitative clinical research. Postdoctoral research is usually supported by clinician scientist fellowship schemes or other post-doctoral support from organisations such as the Department of Health, the Medical Research Council (www.mrc.ac.uk), the Wellcome Trust (www.wellcome.ac.uk), or other charities.

After the postgraduate qualification, some GPs become lecturers. Clinical lectureships provide 50% funding for four years so that GPs may continue research. Senior lectureships lasting five years can lead to becoming a professor. This is funded by the Higher Education Funding Council for England (www.hefce.ac.uk) and the Department of Health (www.dh.gov.uk). GPs with a doctorate may also secure postdoctoral or career scientist fellowships from national funding schemes. If you decide to leave academic general practice and re-enter the field at a later date this is also possible, after negotiation with the organisations involved. *See* Figure 6.1 for some possible ways to enter and develop an academic career.

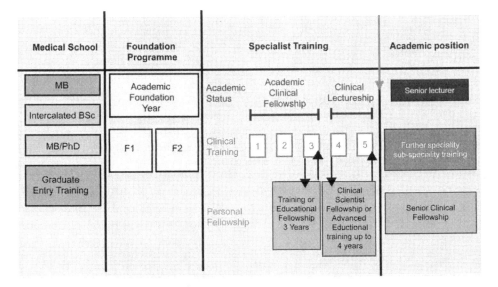

Figure 6.1: The Walport Pathway for Academic Training

Alternative routes

For those who do not follow an official academic path and decide to join later, it is not too late to have an academic career. Since the Walport report, funding opportunities for doctors who want to do research are available, if a doctor can demonstrate an interest in research. If you have an interest in a particular aspect of research or education, it is worth pursuing this by contacting local deaneries, education centres or research departments and finding out how you could fit in within the organisation. Start by developing a research idea and approaching the right people in the department you wish to work with. Do not be afraid to talk to or send an e-mail or letter directly to an academic or clinical fellow you have heard about in the department – if it is the wrong person they are usually happy to help point you towards the right person. Ask previous academic GPs in your area for advice on whom and how to approach people in the relevant department. People will often be willing to support you through the application process, as long as you have sufficient evidence of previous research and academic work. Doing research projects, audits and reflective pieces in journals or health-related magazines can be a way of demonstrating a commitment. This has to go hand in hand with determination and enthusiasm, and the ability to commit to a project for a certain period of time.

Once you have a research project and a department to work with, following the three-year specialist training scheme, you may apply for a two-year academic post combining clinical and academic work and sometimes including a master's degree. Following this fellowship, you can apply for a further academic training fellowship, but because it can be difficult to prepare an application in a short time, the UK Clinical Research Collaboration (UKCRC) and MMC report suggests a one-year additional scheme for GPs during which they can prepare an application for a postdoctoral fellowship.

The portfolio

At all stages in your training, it is worth keeping a portfolio of your achievements, learning experiences, courses, certificates and publications. Trainee doctors are provided with an online or paper portfolio, with assessments by peers and supervisors. Having a portfolio of achievements provides evidence of your continuing professional development and an easy reference for you when applying for jobs. As well as this, your supervisor may wish to see your portfolio as evidence in your supervision sessions. Using the portfolio as a way of recording your achievements, learning experiences, and your goals as you work, will leave you with a good collection of evidence. During your medical education, you will have scheduled meetings with your trainers and supervisors to make sure you are getting the right training – attend these sessions and organise the meetings and agendas for each in advance as these will be on-going and are a useful learning experience. You will learn how to be a good supervisor yourself, and sometimes, how not to be, by attending these sessions. Throughout your career self-appraisal and assessment by others will be part of your on-going learning and can provide very useful personalised feedback on your progress.

Pitfalls in academic general practice

For some, the lack of clinical practice in academic general practice can be a downside. However, if at an early stage you know how much clinical work you wish to undertake, you can try to structure your career this way, to get the right balance. As well as this, keeping up with the multiple roles that are played as an academic and managing time between personal life, clinical work, teaching and research can be demanding. You need a high level of self-discipline and self-motivation as many of these roles will be quite isolated. There are constant pressures to keep to deadlines and juggle the complex needs of patients as well as research. Another pitfall is the lack of contact with other clinicians, leaving you to sometimes feel regarded as the researcher in the 'ivory tower' of primary care, more involved with policy than patients. This can however be avoided, if necessary, by making sure you recognise when the balance is not right, trying to change your commitments accordingly and making sure you continue to have a dialogue with other practitioners on the 'shop-floor'.

My career path: Reflections

At the time of writing, I am a GP registrar and I first experienced an academic post as a Foundation Year 2 doctor. I felt lucky to get a post as it was very competitive to get one. My Foundation Year 2 consisted of the usual posts for a second-year doctor, except for the last four months, which were my academic component. This is a very short time to do much of substance, and as well as that, the post was new, so it was a case of making best use of the post as possible. I was based in a North London general practice for four sessions a week and the rest of the time was spent in the Centre for Aging Population Studies at the Department of Primary Care and Population Sciences (www.ucl.ac.uk/pcps) at the Royal Free and Whittington Hospitals. The exposure to general practice was invaluable, learning the realities of my future career choice and confirming that I had made the right decision. The choice of academic component was relatively flexible. I was given a choice of on-going research opportunities in the Department to get involved in. There were many highly influential and frankly hugely inspiring professors, doctors, researchers and scientists heading important pieces of research relevant to general practice. After looking into the projects underway I met Professor Steve Iliffe, an academic GP involved in medical education and co-director of the Centre for Aging Population Studies.

During that all-too-brief four-month period I started work on two papers, using data collected using the Health Risk Appraisal for Older persons (HRA-O) questionnaire on health behaviours and status (Iliffe, 2007). This research looked into what aspects of preventive care older people do not get access to, and what characteristics of these older people make them less likely to have preventive care checks. I also started research using the same data, on self-efficacy and access to primary care in older people. During my post, I learnt how to use statistics software and became familiar with statistics and research methods. My research at the Centre is on-going, despite officially leaving the department for my next clinical posts, and I have kept in contact with the team there, continuing to learn. During my post, I took every opportunity to learn about the things I was interested in, taking courses in teaching medical students and communication skills, and also held lectures about medical education for GPs. I looked at the Continuing Professional Development spine of the University College London medical school curriculum and helped assess students' progress and the curriculum itself.

During medical school, I had an interest in writing and undertook a BA in Medical Journalism, so I continued to write articles for medically related journals. My, at the time, unconventional choice of doing an intercalated BA in medical journalism at the University of Westminster (www.westminster.ac.uk/schools/media/journalism/ba-medical-journalism) has resulted in writing becoming an important part of my academic activities, having since written a book for patients who have had a stroke (Raymond, 2009) and also coordinating a student essay prize for *Medicine, Conflict and Survival* journal (www.tandf.co.uk/journals/mcs).

I then moved on to a non-academic general practice vocational training scheme in London, continuing my research at the Centre for Aging Population in my own time, and have just started an academic ST4 post. While it is at times difficult to manage all the facets of my clinical work, writing and research, it is a challenge I relish, allowing me a variety of experience while learning skills that interlink with and complement each other. It is an exciting field to be in.

Conclusion

To summarise, academic general practice is what you make of it. You need to have a clear idea that you want to pursue it, as it is not easy (and probably takes years to master the art) to balance the clinical responsibilities you have with the academic. Once you have made that decision, you need to be hard working and self-motivated and constantly reassess your position in terms of work-life balance and research opportunities. The work is very rewarding, especially seeing your research findings put into practice and the students you teach continue to enjoy learning.

Further reading

The following list and references may be helpful if you are looking for more information on how to enter into academic general practice, and will give you an idea of the type of research and teaching that can be part of academic work.

For a guide to academic foundation programmes go to www.foundation programme.nhs.uk

The Association for the Study of Medical Education www.asme.org.uk

National Institute for Health Research's Coordinating Centre for Research Capacity Development www.nccrcd.nhs.uk

Association of Medical Research Charitie www.amrc.org.uk/homepage

UK Research Office www.ukro.ac.uk

UK Federation of Primary Care Research Organisations www.ukf-pcro.org

National Association of Primary Care Educators UK www.napce.net

Journals

Education for Primary Care is the official journal of the UK Association of Programme Directors (UKAPD), the National Association of Primary Care Educators UK and the World Organisation of Family Doctors (WONCA). www.radcliffe-oxford.com/journals/J02_Education_for_Primary_Care

London Journal of Primary Care is a web-based journal for, and by, all those medical and non-medical professionals in primary care in London. www.londonjournalofprimarycare.org.uk

British medical journal www.bmj.com

The Lancet www.thelancet.com

Quality in Primary Care www.radcliffe-oxford.com/journals/J10_Quality_in_Primary_Care

The Journal of Epidemiology and Community Health www.jech.bmj.com

References

HM Treasury. *Science and Innovation: working towards a ten-year investment framework*. London: HMSO; 2004.

Iliffe S, Kharicha K, Harari D, *et al.* Health risk appraisal in older people: Are older people living alone an at risk group? *Brit J Gen Pract.* 2007; **57**(537): 271–276.

Maynard M, Purvis J. Methods, practice and epistemology: the debate about feminism and research. In: Maynard M, Purvis J, editors. *Researching Women's Lives From a Feminist Perspective*. London: Taylor and Francis; 1994, pp. 10–26.

Raymond M. *Coping with Life after Stroke*. London: Sheldon Press; 2009.

Walport M. *Report of the Academic Careers Sub-Committee of Modernising Medical Careers and the UK Clinical Research Collaboration.* London: MMC and the NHS; 2005.

Career profile:

Steve Iliffe

When did you qualify?
I walked into the London MBBS Finals in the summer of 1974 as a qualified doctor. This was possible if you took the exams to be a Licentiate of the Royal College of Physicians and Member of the Royal College of Surgeons. Doing this was not so uncommon at the time, and was enormously reassuring. I was trained on the Central Middlesex GP rotation.

What is your job?
From 1978 to 2007 I worked in general practice in Kilburn, in NW London, starting out as a trainee and ending up as senior partner at Lonsdale Medical Centre. Since 2007 I have been Professor of Primary Care for Older People at University College London, mostly concentrating on research but also spending a session or two each week as a Practice Based Commissioner in Kilburn locality.

Why and how did you choose general practice?
I went to medical school with the intention of becoming a GP, but I do not know exactly where this desire came from. It was not a family tradition, because I was the first person in my family to continue education beyond 16, let alone go to University. During the undergraduate course I was tempted by other specialisms, but not for long.

Where did you work and what did you do?
The first task in the general practice where I worked was to modernise it. That meant having management meetings and documenting decisions, typing referral letters not writing them by hand, sorting out and summarising notes, and hiring a nurse. The receptionists were a problem and had to be turned into a more efficient and less patient-hostile team. Practice income grew when attention was paid to it, the medical team expanded and became more dynamic, and we rapidly ran out of space.

What is the most rewarding aspect of your job?
There were lots of rewards in developing an inner-city general practice. The patient population we served was fascinating, if hard work. We did a nationality count and gave up after 115. I did not meet an Inuit in the time I was there, but I did do a house call to a Tibetan priest in a tower block. Taking on a major teaching commitment enlivened and energised the team. Pushing boundaries made the work exciting – we supported home births in

the eighties, had more than our share of HIV positive patients and set up a drug dependency service in house.

What is the most challenging thing about your job?

The hard part of working in a group is keeping it dynamic without excluding members. All convoys sail at the speed of the slowest ship, and those in the practice wanting to go faster were often frustrated. I am not sure that I got that right all the time.

If you could change one thing about your career what would it be?

I took up academic work early on, in the early eighties, but expanded it when general practice was an uncomfortable place because of the promotion of fund-holding, and the University offered security and sanity. As it happens I moved towards research rather than to teaching, but if I had to serve my time over again I would be biased towards teaching because I think the gains to general practice are greater there.

What do you wish you knew then that you know now?

The claim by general practice to be biopsychosocial medicine is exaggerated. Most GPs know little about either the 'psycho-' or the 'socio-' parts of the job as this is squeezed out of the curriculum. Had I realised that earlier I would have opted for the kind of Masters Degree in primary care that would have filled the gaps, such as a masters in primary care, health psychology or mental health, but being an academic now is a belated attempt to catch up.

Reflective piece: 'Academic general practice'

Surinder Singh

'Those three things, autonomy, complexity and a connection between effort and reward – are, most people agree, the three qualities that work has to have if it is to be satisfying. It is not how much money we make that ultimately makes us happy between nine and five. It's whether our work fulfils us.'

Gladwell, 2008

I'm not sure how I ended up in a small but expanding practice in Deptford. I think I once answered an advert for a single-handed doctor in a practice and as the saying goes, the rest is history. I have now been there for the past 19 years, having qualified nine years previously.

To be honest I think I've taken a portfolio route to where I am, combining teaching at various institutions, clinical practice and other roles as mentor, editorial board member and latterly GMC performance assessor. It is an interesting mix and no two days are alike.

I relish a varied working week, for example, seeing patients, writing, research, attending committee meetings and, of course, teaching. I really started wholesale teaching at London Lighthouse – post vocational training – when it was my job as a medical officer (current equivalent would be a GP Registrar or ST3) to try and relay important information to patients, carers and family members about HIV and AIDS. The conditions were new back then and lots of myths had fuelled inaccurate information and we saw it as our job to try to reverse this trend. I was told at the time that I did it well, conversed in a way which was person-friendly and that I kept my composure. My role as a medical officer was to welcome patients into the unit and plan their stay, whether for symptom-control, rehabilitation or respite.

I had known for a long time that I could not do full time clinical practice, for me the 5 days seemed excessive and other interests would be stifled out (see later). This is an important lesson for those still trying to work out their career – sometimes knowing what you don't want to do is a way to finding your ultimate direction. My HIV and AIDS interests paid dividends, for example being invited to conferences and the occasional talk, which boosted confidence and gave me an insight into the 'academic world'. I liked it.

I went on to undertake an MSc in Medical Anthropology which I enjoyed. My big regret about this is that I'm not sure I have put any of it into practice – except I would like to think that my understanding of things 'cultural' is perhaps a bit more developed than most.

I currently lead on the iBSc at University College London (UCL, 2010) which is great fun but it has its moments. It is quite a responsibility ensuring that all proceeds well for students to attain their degrees. The most satisfying part is to see students flourish and excel, often from very junior status – for example second-year medical students – through to submitting their dissertations and then on to presenting at small conferences. Such is the value and quality of their original research.

What works very well in all of this is that practice integrates with the academia and I don't get bogged down too much during the week. Unfortunately sometimes there is conflict with both practice (my partners are understanding but there is always a limit) and the University (exam schedules are usually non-negotiable) though it is ultimately up to me to resolve this as best I can.

Latterly, I work with the General Medical Council as a performance assessor – this is fascinating but in many ways presents an interesting reflexivity about one's own practice. I am constantly thinking when performance-assessing the doctors in front of us; how would I react in similar circumstances? Would I have written my notes like that? Would I have handled such a patient in this way? Ultimately, this is about 'protecting patients'…and in many ways is another facet of a public service – in which I feel privileged to be able to contribute.

Working part-time in practice has its moments. When I'm there, it really is 'full-on' – Tuesday, my 'first day of the week' is seeing patients in the morning, followed by the practice weekly clinical meeting and then afternoon catch-up with an evening surgery. The last patient is usually booked in at 7.30pm. I've not always done this, but have done over the previous year – partially in response to the threat of another practice opening up just down the corridor!

A good Tuesday is when I have time to catch-up, e.g. talk to our manager. A bad one – like last week, when a genuine emergency precipitated a home-visit, I returned for a bite to eat, and then failed to complete the repeat prescriptions before seeing an 'extra' (patient) all before surgery 'officially' started at 5pm.

I think clinical practice is getting harder – though I am not sure I know why. Is it the burden of looking after a medium-sized practice in an area where nothing is certain and the constant upheaval and change that seems to characterise healthcare in the UK? Or maybe it is 28 years of clinical practice – nothing more and nothing less. One thing of which I am certain – the mixture of clinical work and academia works well for me most of the time, though I acknowledge that this calls for flexibility all round, both from the University and the practice.

References

Gladwell M. *The Three Lessons of Joe Flom. Outliers – the story of success.* London: Penguin Books; 2008.

UCL. *Intercalated BSc in Primary Health Care.* 2010. [Online]. Available at: www.ucl.ac.uk/pcph/education/undergrad/bsc_pc/index.htm (accessed 31 May 2010).

CHAPTER 7

Professional development

Andrew Dicker

Does professional development refer to a professional way of developing or the development of a professional? The latter idea is more appealing. The Shorter Oxford English Dictionary offers various definitions of development which include: 'a gradual unfolding', 'a fuller working out of the details of anything', 'the growth of what is in the germ' and 'growth from within'. When applied to a professional as a person these processes acquire an organic sense.

Another way of thinking about what professional development means is learning. Learning is constant and organic. Every experience provides something new which is capable of expanding our perspective. For experience or discovery to become part of our learning, a process of reflection is necessary to understand the meaning of what has happened and how it relates to our thoughts and actions. It is fortunate that the ability and desire to learn is innate in the human species. The means by which we implement this ability to make it function in a practical way is what developing the professional person is all about.

Learning styles

The industry which has grown around the need and compulsion not just to learn, but to be seen to be learning, is increasingly complex and regulated. Learning is an intensely personal process and does not readily lend itself to contemporary ways of achieving it, prescribed by someone else, whose needs are not necessarily consonant with our own. For learning to be effective, it needs to be done in the knowledge of what style of learning is personal to the learner. There are ways to identify and label learning styles by completing questionnaires. Rather like psychometric testing such methods tend to confirm what we already know. Some people like learning on their own in libraries or on the internet. Others thrive in groups. Didactically delivered lectures suit some people but bore others. A little reflection will usually tell us what we need to know about ourselves in this respect and a little more reflection, preferably with someone else, will tell us a great deal about our individual learning needs. So once we discover how we learn best and what we need to learn, the rest is easy.

Developmental hedonism

It is a characteristic of all learning and development – 'the growth of what is in the germ' – that unless it is enjoyable, it is unlikely to be effective. This is a point which is generally not sufficiently emphasised. A motivated learner will rapidly cease to learn and may even become demotivated, if the experience of learning is not an enjoyable one. Developmental hedonism is a prerequisite ingredient in any learning environment. Learning, in any context, ideally should be something to which it is possible to look forward. Anticipation of the process, or structured session, predisposes to the enthusiasm of the learners and the desire to derive something unique from the experience. Everyone has their own recollections of memorable learning because it was enjoyable. The reason it was enjoyable was because the experience involved some critical discovery of something not known before and the intrinsic sense of success which accompanies the growth of knowledge or experience.

Training to be a General Practitioner

For many years, the professional development of general practitioners (GPs) has been through exposure to clinical work in hospitals and general practices, increasingly the latter. Training to be a GP takes a minimum of three years, four years in a handful of training schemes, and may soon take five years, mostly in practice. Although the experience of professional development in the hospital setting is often a challenging and interesting time, many trainees find that after four months in a hospital specialty setting that they have learnt all they are going to learn, which is relevant to primary care, in the context of the particular attachment. While there is always more to learn, there is also the developmental process of discovering what it is most important to learn, on the trajectory of training. So, it is entirely appropriate that most of the time spent in training should be with patients in primary care.

The main transformation which doctors undergo during the trainee years is when they embark on the practice-based part of the training. A lot of hospital-based 'history-taking' habits need to be unlearnt and a new way of talking to patients adopted. The GP consultation has been characterised as an 'ethical conversation' by teachers of systemic supervision. An ethical conversation happens in a meeting between patient and doctor. It is devoid of judgementalism and attempts to place the patient's problem in the wider context of their life, using a systemic approach, and sharing an understanding of both the patient's and the doctor's perspective. It entails developing the art of listening.

Training doctors to be GPs is undertaken by experienced GPs who are approved and re-approved to be trainers every three years by the local postgraduate deanery. There is no doubt that the experience of seeing and managing patients is the most useful activity in the development of GPs, as long as there are boundaries in place to prevent the exploitation of the over-zealous trainee. The day-to-day work is supplemented by regular one-to-one supervision with the trainer where any subject can be addressed, from cases which the trainee finds confusing, to more formal teaching of subjects identified by assessment of the trainee's learning needs. This is an apprenticeship model in which the relationship of trainer to trainee is an important part of professional development and unique to the training of GPs. It is important that trainee and trainer are happy to spend a significant part of the week in each other's company. A dysfunctional relationship between learner and supervisor can be disastrous. For this reason, the way in which different training schemes organise the placement of trainees is an important part of the preparation which should seek to avoid 'mismatches'.

The GP curriculum

As in all specialties a curriculum exists which GP trainees must demonstrate that they have covered during their training (*see* Chapter 2: General practice specialty training). The curriculum was, and continues to be, developed by the Royal College of General Practitioners (RCGP). It is very long and rather repetitive. Curriculum coverage during training is facilitated by the obligatory use of an e-portfolio, personal to every trainee, but accessible to trainers and other educators in a supervisory role. In addition to a fixed number of supervised clinical activities, in which competence must be demonstrated, the e-portfolio allows the trainee to record individual, reflective experiences which contribute to learning. Each piece of recorded learning contributes to coverage of one or other area of the curriculum. The trainee's supervisor is able to validate the entry by electronically endorsing it with a particular professional competence to which the recorded experience relates. Over time, the trainee is able to demonstrate coverage of the entire curriculum and acquisition of the competencies which will enable independent practice by the end of training.

A more vibrant activity, to which all GP trainees have had access for many years, is the educational programme which runs in parallel to their other professional activities. These programmes are provided nationally by the postgraduate deaneries. They are run by experienced GPs who have an interest in education. The sessions happen once a week and the trainees are expected to attend, service commitments permitting. These weekly sessions are unique to general practice training. They provide a sense of professional cohesion among a community of highly motivated doctors, the majority of whom have succeeded in being recruited to a training scheme of their choice, in preparation for their chosen specialty. The potential to capitalise on the enthusiasm of these learning groups is obvious.

The way in which these programmes are provided are unique and idiosyncratic. The content of the programmes is dependent on the approach of the programme directors, who are empowered by the deaneries to provide what they believe to be educational in the broadest sense. In some programmes, there may be a series of sessions designed prescriptively to assist the trainees to cover the curriculum. In other programmes, the content may be designed by the trainees themselves, with the guidance of the programme directors, and run in an overtly learner-centred, interactive style. In particular, the latter model predisposes to the inclusion of a broad range of topics which may include politics, ethics, humanities, management, leadership, medicine and anything else which may contribute to the development of the trainees. Traditionally, the sessions are run as a form of group learning and emphasis is put on group cohesion, which predisposes to the functional conduct of the group, and aids learning.

The role of the programme directors is primarily to deliver the educational programme but they also have a significant pastoral role, not least because they relate to the trainees for the whole duration of their training. The directors have a degree of authority in the running of the training schemes and relate to and support the hospital doctors and trainers, but are responsible to the deanery, not the hospital trusts. The independence which this model creates is important in that it allows the directors to handle problems which may arise, in the individual progress of trainees, in an unencumbered and unbiased way. They are able to be the unprejudiced advocates for the trainees, should the need arise.

Balint groups

One of the most common activities which go on in the trainee groups are case discussions. The groups are an obvious environment where discussion among peers about difficult or stuck cases can be held in a non-judgemental atmosphere. One of the more sophisticated models of case discussion are Balint groups. The focus of Balint group discussions is the relationship between patient and doctor. Ideally, the groups are led by accredited Balint group leaders and have no more than about ten members.

The discussion is begun by the leader asking the group 'Who has a case?' A doctor will present a case without reference to notes. The cases tend to be complex. When the case is finished, the group members are invited to ask factual questions to clarify the detail. The presenting doctor is then absented, metaphorically, from the ensuing discussion. The group members are encouraged to use imagination and fantasy to explore the context of the case, the feelings which it aroused in both patient and doctor and how the relationship between doctor and patient affected the process of the consultation. The clinical detail of the case is de-emphasised. Towards the end of the discussion, the presenting doctor is invited to 'rejoin' the group and observe how or why the discussion helped to move the case on, or not. This approach is made unique by being a demedicalised case discussion between doctors.

Reflection

Training to be a GP is a long formative process. There is much encouragement to reflect on experience. Reflection, in this context, is a process of assimilating both new learning, and the significance of things which have happened, to give them meaning. For structured learning, or things learnt through experience, to be meaningful they need to be relevant to practice. How newly acquired knowledge can be applied to practice is something which the process of reflection can facilitate.

Acquiring the habit of reflection is one of the building blocks of professional development and has great relevance in the context of appraisal. Among other things the process of reflection entails demonstrating a critical approach to the subject in question and the capacity in the learner to be self-critical. Revalidation requires doctors to be able to demonstrate not just evidence of learning, but how learning can contribute to, or change, professional behaviour. Appraisal is the means to this end. The formative learning which takes place during the years training to be a GP has the potential to create learning habits which will be essential to independent practice. Far from being the end of learning, completion of training is the stage from which self-directed learning can subsequently flourish.

Professional development after training

Much of the structured learning which takes place during GP training happens in groups. Historically, GPs have been proponents of learning in groups which create a non-didactic, interactive learning environment. The habit is frequently perpetuated into the early years of independent practice in the form of young practitioner groups (*see* Chapter 4: Locum and out-of-hours work, for an example). These are self-directed groups of recently trained doctors who are able to support one another, academically and pastorally, through the early years of independent practice. The work environment to which GPs in training are exposed is relatively protected. Because training practices are re-approved by their deanery every three years, the organisational and clinical standards must be maintained. For most GPs, the first encounter with the world of general practice, where training does not take place, is on the occasion of their first appointment to a job, which will often be part-time and probably salaried. It is a paradoxically isolated time suddenly separated from the supportive training environment.

Mentoring is another activity which has been adopted widely by postgraduate organisations. It can be used as a means to the end of optimising the potential of GPs and finding ways for doctors to resolve problems which arise in the early years of independent practice. It is probably true that everyone should try mentoring, while acknowledging that it is neither therapy nor the right approach for everyone. It entails a one to one opportunity to reflect on both successes and difficulties which arise, in a professional context, with an empathetic peer, skilled in the art of mentoring. It is not without risks, and while it has been a useful activity for many doctors, should not be seen as a solution to problems which it is not designed to solve. For some doctors, it may be one of the means to the end of achieving 'a gradual unfolding; a fuller working out of the details of anything' in the rich armament of developmental opportunities.

There is a bewildering array of postgraduate educational events on offer around the UK. Somewhere during the years of training it is to be hoped, perhaps in vain, that a sense of discernment is instilled among the learners. The wheat of postgraduate education needs to be distinguished from the chaff, so the 'growth of what is in the germ' can truly flourish and not be distracted by the commodification of professional development. Clearly, there is profit to be made from the provision of courses in almost anything, in exchange for a fee, and the provision of the vacuous 'certificate of attendance.' The pursuit of postgraduate education must be approached critically without losing the fundamental need to sustain a sense of enjoyment in the process.

Learning needs

Learning needs are always the key to the direction learning should follow. Specialists logically hone their specialist skills and knowledge. GPs, being generalists, are faced with a paradox. They complete a specialist training course but are, by definition, generalists. Within most generalists there is a germ of specialism and it is to this that most GPs will gravitate in the selection of which aspect of their professional selves to develop.

Dermatologically interested GPs know more than they need to know about skin diseases but still sign up for the dermatology updates; GPs versed in medical ethics go to more ethics conferences; the GP paediatricians return to the paediatric courses and so on. There has always been a tendency to neglect real learning needs because it is easier, perhaps more enjoyable, to do more of what we are good at already rather than challenge the margins of generalist expertise.

For the concept of professional development to have meaning, the identification of learning needs is critical, particularly in the face of the target driven and trivial box-ticking culture which pervades primary care in the NHS. Truly independent and self-directed professional development is a cornerstone of professionalism. It requires a particular sort of courage and humility to acknowledge the existence of a hiatus in expertise or understanding. In every consultation there is an element of uncertainty. While uncertainty may create discomfort it is also a prolific source of unmet learning needs. A willingness to seek the reason for whatever has created a sense of uncertainty, and the capacity to be self-critical, are essential ingredients of a professional approach to reflective, professional development.

Another way of describing the process of professional development is as the thing which the life-long learner does. The ideal product of training schemes for general practice is the doctor devoted to enlarging the learning acquired in the early years of practice. The ability to work independently as a doctor is unique to GPs. The ability to work in a team is another prerequisite of professionalism but independence, in the sense of not working in a hierarchy, but making the interest of the patient the first concern of the professionally confident doctor, is intrinsic to the role of GPs.

Experience

The accrual of experience is intrinsic to working as a GP and is one of its greatest rewards. Experience is a part of the outcome of professional development and is considerably undervalued in the contemporary climate of evidence and guidelines. Experience, as a professional attribute, had a hard time during the last decade of the 20th century with the emergence of evidence-based practice as the gold standard of how to practice. Sackett coined the aphorism 'experience is the best excuse for ignorance' at the height of the evidence-based euphoria of the 1990s (Sackett *et al*, 1981). With hindsight, this notion is shallow and reductionist. The value of experience is inestimable to those who possess it. Experience contributes an essential dimension to the way GPs consult and is acquired through the process of professional development and reflection. But more importantly the potential of the continuity of care, which is unique to the way GPs practice, underpins the value and practical implementation of the wisdom with which experience endows those who possess it.

Evidence can be defined as the expression of the aggregated information concerning populations from randomised controlled trials. As Petr Skrabanek pointed out at the end of the 1980s, before the 'evidence-basers' caught the headlines, it is illogical to apply the quantitative results of research from populations to individuals because they are not the same thing (Skrabanek and McCormick, 1989). Although 'evidence' is the main source of objective information which informs the guidelines which tell doctors how to manage particular medical conditions, every GP knows that it does not always work. The unique quality of experience, acquired through practice, and the pastoral knowledge of individuals in a community, provides both the recognition of when guidelines may or may not be sufficient, and why.

Therefore, it becomes evident that whatever external sources of professional development and learning may be appropriate, the central component of the process is doing the work of general practice and understanding the potential of every consultation as a source of learning. This is why an understanding of what is happening in a consultation, the process, is so important through participation in such activities as Balint groups. Professional development is not just about knowing more and more medicine. It is also about knowing more and more about the people who come to see their GP, and the GPs coming to know more about themselves, and why it is that no two consultations are alike.

Actively cultivating a sense of curiosity is fundamental to the development of an understanding of why one consultation feels rewarding and another becomes a source of frustration or distress. So, the acknowledgement of the existence of feelings in both patient and doctor, and their effect upon the interaction, is an essential part of professional development. This is also key to developing a systemic approach to the process of consulting. While some of this can be learnt from a variety of sources designed for the purpose, it is the growing understanding of the self which becomes the main source of the real development of the professional person. The acquisition of experience matters more than anything else. It is a happy coincidence that all GPs can achieve this just by doing the job!

And finally

Professional development, as a necessary activity for GPs, is likely to have as many ways of being interpreted as there are people actively involved in doing it. I would propose that, in the pursuit of one plausible outcome for the process, learners at any stage in their development should construe the process as the means to the end of acquiring the courage **to be able** to exercise their clinical judgement. Courage is a necessary virtue for GPs to possess in the face of guidelines which may seem to conflict with what is the least harmful course of action for the patient.

Further sources and reading

The King's Fund: http://www.kingsfund.org.uk/ provide a number of relevant publications and also arrange workshops and courses.

The Balint Society: http://balint.co.uk/ produce a regular journal and run a number of courses and groups across the UK.

The Royal College of General Practice: http://www.rcgp.org.uk/ produce a regular journal (the *British Journal of General Practice*) which contains essays and reflections about professional practice on its back pages. There is also a journal for associates in training called 'InnovAiT'. The RCGP runs a number of courses, seminars and conferences.

The RCGP 'First 5' programme has been specifically developed to support GP trainees in the first 5 years after graduation and run several events to support professional development: http://www.rcgp.org.uk/new_professionals/first5.aspx.

Your local Deanery may also offer courses to support professional development in a variety of ways. John Launer, for example, runs a number of courses and seminars at the Tavistock and London Deanery on clinical supervision for teachers in primary care: http://www.faculty.londondeanery.ac.uk/super vision-skills-for-clinical-teachers.

Narrative-based Primary Care: a practical guide by John Launer.

From General Practice to Primary Care: the industrialization of family medicine by Steve Iliffe.

The Reflective Practitioner: how professionals think in action by Donald Schon

Medicine and Literature: The Doctor's Companion to the Classics by Iona Heath and John Salinsky.

References

Sackett D, Haynes RB, Guyatt GH, *et al. Clinical Epidemiology: A Basic Science for Clinical Medicine*. London: Little, Brown & Co; 1981.

Skrabanek P, McCormick J. *Follies and Fallacies in Medicine* (2nd edn). Whithorn: Tarragon Press; 1989.

Reflective piece: 'What Balint did for me'

John Salinsky

When I first started in general practice, I was gratified to find that, after a few months, I began to develop my own little flock of patients. These were people who actually came to me by choice and regarded me as 'their doctor'. Some of these were people with whom I had scored a lucky diagnostic success; others I just got along with very well and they seemed to like me too.

But there were also patients who brought out the worst in me. They made me feel irritable or even angry. I would try to contain these negative feelings, but every so often they would escape. Before I knew it, the consultation would have gone out of control. I would hear a voice, very like my own, saying outrageous things like: 'Why don't you listen? You're just wasting my time' or 'It's all your own fault', or 'Of course you don't need an antibiotic. Who is the doctor here, me or you?'. These unprofessional outbursts may have contained a few home truths but they didn't make me feel good. This was not the way it was supposed to be. I thought of myself as a nice doctor.

Although the patients were offended they didn't always desert me. Some seemed to stay on just for the pleasure of provoking me. Requests for 'unnecessary' home visits were a frequent irritant that made me flare up angrily on the phone; there were a lot of home visits in those days. The patient was usually an elderly lady on her own.

> 'Why can't you come to the surgery?'
>
> 'I'm not well enough.'
>
> 'Of course you are, you've had that pain for months. Years. And if I do come out, there will be nothing I can do. As I've told you a hundred times, *it's all due to stress.*'
>
> 'Please come, doctor. I can't stand it anymore. I'll have to call for an ambulance.'
>
> 'Oh all right, then (grinding my teeth) I'll be there in half an hour. But you're just wasting my time.'
>
> 'Thank you, doctor.'

So, I would go round, end up accepting a cup of tea and a piece of cake, and not feel too bad. Until the next time!

When a Balint group came along I was happy to join. I had heard about them from my elder brother who had been a member of one of the great man's early groups. I was expecting to learn some psychotherapeutic skills to apply to the patients I liked; but I soon found myself talking about the ones who drove me into a rage. It was a relief to tell my tales from the front line and to be able to see the funny side. My fellow group members were so sympathetic; they had all been there themselves, even if their reactions were not as incendiary as mine. In the discussion, people made interesting suggestions about what was going on between the patient and me. Some of the old ladies were clearly reminding me of my mother. Other patients seemed to represent a side of myself that I would rather not know about. These included the ones with insatiable and contemptible desires for a forbidden prescription; a narcotic or a tranquilliser; or merely an antibiotic. And yet I too knew what it was like to be unable to resist temptation. Or to feel denied the one thing I felt I needed. I began to see that it was possible to see things from the patient's point of view and to find something to like in the most disordered of personalities.

I didn't altogether stop flying into rages. But it happened less often. And I also found that I could apologise and ask the patient if we could start again. Sometimes when we did that, the relationship became better than I could have foreseen. On one occasion, I had been called to do a home visit by a woman who was having problems with her schizoid teenage son. He was seeing a psychiatrist and was on medication. He didn't seem too bad to me and yet she wanted me to get him admitted as an emergency. I refused this unreasonable request without quite appreciating the distress and disappointment that she was feeling. In the end, I stormed out of the house and slammed the door behind me. Fifty yards down the road, I thought, 'No this won't do. I feel terrible'. I ran back to the house, and knocked on the door. She opened it at once and, without a word, we fell into each other's arms in silent reconciliation. It could only happen in general practice.

Reflective piece: 'When it happens to us'

Anna Denshuck

How do we cope with illness when it happens to us? Does it make a difference to how we practice? Certainly, I've noticed that I feel more sympathetic towards patients presenting with colds when I've just had one. But have you ever considered how you would cope if, unexpectedly, you were sitting in the patient's chair, receiving a life threatening diagnosis? Perhaps we think it won't happen to us, or perhaps we can't even process the thought, as it is too difficult to cope with. Perhaps it's something that we inwardly fear, or perhaps it's none of these.

I clearly remember worrying that I had various illnesses as a medical student, matching relevant diagnostic features to my previously trivial concerns, which then diminished once we moved onto the next topic. I assume that, subconsciously, I continued to worry about my health, because later I had a recurring dream whilst practising hospital medicine. I dreamt I was diagnosed with lung cancer and given only a few days to live. I was viewing a chest X-ray with a consultant, as if in a teaching session. He used a pointer to tap the X-ray, 'What does this show?' he said. I suddenly realised that it was an X-ray of my own lungs and there was a shadow on it…

Fast-forward five years. Life interrupted. One morning I noticed a small breast lump whilst moisturizing, surely just a fibro-adenoma, I thought. My GP seemed a bit cagey about what she thought it was; I had been expecting a brush off; after all, I was only 28 years old; I didn't even qualify for the two-week referral according to the NICE guidelines (I later discovered that she too had had breast cancer at a young age). Soon I was attending for my results following triple assessment. To my shock and horror, my consultant told me I had breast cancer. I couldn't hear anything else he said after that, my life seemed to shatter into pieces around me; I couldn't find anything to hold onto, it was all slipping away. I assumed that I would be dead within weeks.

So how did I cope? Lots of people said, 'you're coping really well', which felt odd because I wasn't thinking about coping well, just about surviving. Some days I wanted to scream and shout at the injustice of it all, others, it was all I could muster to get out of bed to face the fear, but the awareness was always there that my emotions, no matter how strong, couldn't change the outcome. Of course, there can be very low times, and depression cannot always be prevented by will alone.

I found that focusing on the positive aspects helped me; 'I'm lucky I don't have to have a mastectomy, only a lumpectomy', 'I'm lucky it's not spread to the lymph nodes', 'I'm lucky its oestrogen-receptor negative as that means I can have IVF to preserve some embryos' (without thinking too hard about the fact that prognosis is worse for oestrogen-receptor negative cancers). I also had a lot of help and support from my GP, not least in seeing her pregnant shortly after my diagnosis, proving in front of my eyes, that there could be life after breast cancer, brilliant counselling at the practice, telephone support set up by the breast cancer care website and participation in a local young women's breast cancer support group. Prior to this, I had underestimated how powerful support groups can be. It does not suit everyone, but it was through this group I met a friend in a similar situation, and it is her friendship that has had the biggest impact on my psychological wellbeing. Having someone to share the unpleasant experiences with, who doesn't pity you, and can laugh with you, is more helpful than any counselling. Plus, thankfully, there are great medical and surgical treatments for breast cancer, so my prognosis is actually very much better than my initial perception of it. Of course, this is much easier to rationalise having passed the 5-year survival or recurrence mark, as well as having had the good fortune to start a family of my own.

So, does practising general practice feel different afterwards? The answer is 'yes and no'. Spending more than one year as a patient, regularly attending the chemotherapy suite, radiotherapy and many other appointments, does sap confidence. It is important not to underestimate the feeling of vulnerability on going back to work. I was fortunate that my training practice was very supportive and allowed me to go back part-time. Some of my most liberating and fulfilling experiences since returning to practice have involved sharing my cancer diagnosis with patients who have been recently diagnosed. A connection like a live-wire seems to crackle between us and a great sigh of being understood (or just heard?) emits from my patient. Initially, I was reluctant to do this; the experience was just too raw. I also knew I needed to have the confidence and ability to keep it professional.

Ultimately, the whole experience has enhanced my understanding of so many things: specific illnesses, specific treatments, being a patient, the frustrations of being a pawn in the hospital system, among others. However, one could argue that many other life experiences do this too. Then, on the other hand, the job I have gone back to is essentially the same, the patients' needs are unchanged; it is me who has changed.

Beforehand, I had been concerned that I might find myself less tolerant of minor complaints, but this hasn't been the case. I have a new awareness that has enabled me to offer support in situations where previously I may not even have recognised the issues.

If there is one thing I hope to convey, it is that although we are all likely to face difficult personal circumstances at some point in our career, this will have its own unique relevance to general practice in terms of our understanding, awareness and ability to support our patients.

CHAPTER 8

Teaching in general practice

Sophie Park

Introduction

Teaching embraces expertise both in a particular *topic* and in its *delivery* in order to facilitate learning. This chapter will focus mainly on the latter. Teaching is of course likely to impact on your practice through motivations to keep up-to-date about particular topic areas. However, in devoting time to development of the teaching *process*, you are also likely to benefit students, patients and yourself as practitioner in other relevant ways, as you begin to make more explicit connections between elements of your professional identity and practice. As a GP (or GP-to-be), you have a particularly privileged position in being able to draw on extensive training in consulting skills. Doctor in Latin actually means 'teacher' (OED, 2010), highlighting many of the similarities between consulting and teaching. The GMC now recognises teaching as an essential element of the role of a doctor (GMC, 2009). The extent and type of this involvement will vary according to your preference and arising opportunities, but I hope to outline some of the generic qualities required of any teaching in general practice.

Many specialities within medicine still have no formal route to support development for teachers within their field (BMA, 2006). General practice however, certainly at postgraduate level, has a well-established and generally excellent set of processes to help those interested in teaching nurture the necessary reflective expertise and acquisition of appropriate knowledge and skills, rooted in the model of apprenticeship. The utilisation of GPs within undergraduate teaching has expanded hugely over the last decade, with GPs adopting a variety of educational roles in medical schools including: practice-based teaching in general practice and specialty placements; professional development programmes; mentoring; and academic positions. In this chapter, I hope to share with you a flavour of both the more formal routes required in order to get involved in teaching, as well as some more informal suggestions to begin developing your teaching practice.

Where to start?

Before deciding how you wish to shape your career in relation to teaching, it is worth spending some time thinking about *you*. Where do you aspire to be in ten years? Do you wish to be a practitioner with an active involvement in practice-based teaching, or extend your teaching role within other institutions or forums? For undergraduate teaching, this might be a university; at postgraduate level, perhaps a role within a deanery or other advisory or assessment body. Would you like to focus on teaching at undergraduate level, postgraduate or combine both? Would you like to get involved in research about medical education? Your interests may change with time, but these questions will help inform your choice about which path is currently most suited to you and consequently, which areas you might focus on for development.

There are many levels of involvement available to the teacher in general practice. The vast majority of GP teachers will be involved in practice-based education. This might be as a trainer for specialist trainees, a supervisor for foundation doctors or Out-of-Hours trainees, or a tutor for undergraduate students. Some of the examples in this chapter focus on undergraduate teaching, but the qualities and elements illustrated are relevant to teaching in most areas of general practice education, whoever the learner. While most GP teachers' involvement is at a practical level, some might wish to become involved in other aspects of general practice education, such as management and organisation, or research and these are discussed below. Whatever your planned trajectory, your first step is likely to be that you become involved in hands-on teaching. As you develop as a teacher and meet others within your local community, you will hopefully begin to forge a pathway best suited to you.

How much will I get paid?

Payment for teaching will vary and there are, of course, a huge number of benefits for the practice aside from financial gain (*see* Box 8.1). There have been moves over recent years to improve payment for teaching by clinicians to introduce an element of parity between the two activities. If, therefore, you are teaching within your capacity as a GP, there is usually a reasonable associated income, although this will vary according to the number of service appointments you will be expected to achieve during your teaching sessions. Teaching within general practice usually generates a reasonable income to allow a practice to provide the same, if not more service appointments as a result. If you are teaching in your role as 'generic educator' rather than 'GP', the payment may vary more widely. Most academic posts for GP educators, depending on their seniority, receive a similar salary to their clinical equivalent sessions.

Box 8.1: Benefits of teaching for practices

➤ The practice becomes recognised as a 'teaching practice', often bringing extra status and respect from patients.

➤ Teaching can help clinicians keep up-to-date in an enjoyable and interactive way.

➤ Patients will often enjoy involvement in teaching, benefitting from the enthusiasm and extra time available from trainees.

➤ Teaching might generate income for additional facilities within the practice.

➤ Teaching can help to vary GPs working week and prevent burn out.

➤ Teaching involvement can nurture inter-professional relationships within the practice.

➤ Teaching will generate income for the practice to replace, if not enhance service provision.

➤ Involvement in teaching, attending related training events etc., can help reduce individuals' feelings of isolation and also build relationships with neighbouring practices, with many other positive consequences.

How do I professionalise as a teacher?

Before drawing upon my own experience with teachers and learners to discuss some practical ways to develop your teaching role, this section will describe the various possible *qualifications* in medical education which might be relevant for a GP teacher. It should, however, be emphasised that most teachers begin by getting involved in teaching *delivery*. They may or may not then decide to pursue a commitment to further qualifications in medical education. This section aims to provide some information to support those choosing a course or qualifications, should this feel the right path for you. There are a number of courses available, some of which are listed at the end of this chapter. Please also *see* Chapter 6: Academic general practice, for a discussion of higher degrees more broadly relevant to primary care.

Many GPs begin their teaching careers in undergraduate education. This requires enthusiasm and responsiveness to feedback, but as yet, no specific qualifications. Many teachers will, however, attend courses as part of their professional development, in addition to events run by the specific university.

A foundation or Out-of-Hours supervisor, will usually be required to do an introductory course to teaching and familiarise themselves with the relevant curriculum, usually facilitated by deaneries over two to three days. Most deaneries now require all those wishing to become a trainer to complete a certificate in clinical education. Programmes, such as the Teaching Improvement Project System (TIPS) or the Introduction to Teaching in Primary Care (ITTPC), available through some universities and deaneries, often form the first components towards a certificate in clinical education within a particular institution. These courses often offer 'practical tips' for teaching and ground this in some theory and reflection relating to your teaching practice. A certificate in clinical education usually takes about one year to complete and is the equivalent of a PGCE held by most primary and secondary school teachers. To extend this further, a second year of study will often convert your certificate to a Diploma qualification, then after completion of a dissertation, a Masters degree.

Box 8.2: Questions to ask staff and existing students before embarking on a particular course

➤ Where does the course take place?
➤ Does it involve weekends, holidays or evenings?
➤ Will I need to negotiate time out of clinical responsibilities to attend teaching or complete written work?
➤ Who will fund the course?
➤ Will I need to adjust personal-life responsibilities and are my surrounding family or friends prepared to support this?
➤ How structured is the course and when are deadlines for written work?
➤ What proportion of the course is attendance or virtual learning?
➤ What facilities are available?
➤ What tutor support is available?

If you wish to be a trainer, supervising ST3 doctors (also referred to as registrars), do make contact with your local deanery before embarking upon a particular route. They may have an existing course specifically orientated to clinical education in primary care, or may accept a similar qualification from a different institution. It is often useful to become acquainted with other trainers in the area and studying together for the certificate is one way of forming these local networks and connections. Once a GP has successfully completed the course, the local deanery will do a 'practice visit' to assess if your practice facilities and procedures provide an appropriate environment for learners. These inspections are the 'gold standard' for involvement in education and are accepted by foundation schools and undergraduate departments, who usually complete similar, but more limited inspections of practices not currently involved in specialist level training. Deanery approval is usually refreshed at three yearly intervals. It may take some time after this practice approval to actually be assigned a trainee, as vocational training programmes are planned many months in advance and are additionally dependent on funding and hospital posts.

You may have other motivations for pursuing professional development in education: perhaps a passionate personal interest in a particular field, or a desire to know more of the theory to inform your teaching practice. Equally, you may have more strategic reasons to acquire a postgraduate qualification such as increased recognition of power or status in your institution, facilitating a change in role or promotion. It is crucial then to match these needs with the course you choose. Many GPs enjoy delivering teaching within their practices. Others wish to extend this role further becoming 'academic GPs', dedicating a number of sessions to a particular undergraduate or postgraduate institution. Traditionally, academics fall into two camps; that of 'researcher' and that of the 'teacher'. Although there is often overlap between the two in many academic roles, issues around associated status, promotion and recognition are complex. These often reflect priorities of particular institutions towards either experiential knowledge, acquired through or in relation to practice, or more research-related theoretical, specialist knowledge. Many post specifications in undergraduate and postgraduate academic roles now include evidence of a higher degree and contribution to the research literature. Recent frameworks for rewarding university departments' activity have also focussed on production of research in high impact journals, rather than valuing teaching activity and general academic citizenship (e.g. contributing to management meetings, teaching and mentoring students, maintaining effective relationships with staff and colleagues, responding to requests for careers advice and developing assessment and curricula), although some teaching posts are exempt from these research-orientated performance targets.

Many teachers wishing to extend their role in organisational or management posts have, therefore, also had to develop their research expertise. This often has explicit benefits for their teaching, increasing their familiarity with a particular area of literature and developing general approaches using critical thinking. It does, however, often mean that academic GPs need at some point to do some research in order to gain promotion in their relevant field. This might be achieved through a small scale research project, or perhaps completion of a Masters, or Doctoral level qualification, such as an MD,

PhD or EdD. All but the last can be done in a clinical specialty, but all can be done in areas of education relating to a medical context. There are a variety of postgraduate programmes available. Each represents its own currency in different contexts, but all represent enormous personal investments of time, tenacity and money. Courses differ in their orientation, some focusing on integration of teaching experience and theory, whereas others are specifically designed to extend participants' research involvement. The latter requires careful attention to the type of research methodologies to be explored. Many educational courses, for example, will broaden your experience to include sociological, historical, philosophical and political perspectives, in addition to the more familiar positivist approaches used in most medical research.

Deciding between doctoral level qualifications again depends very much upon personal motivations, strengths and areas for development. An MD can usually be achieved by those wishing to extend a Masters level project, but offers less potential for supervision than a PhD. A PhD, again requiring independent study, might take three years full-time or five part-time. It usually involves an application with an already well-formed research proposal and choice of two relevant supervisors. It could, in this context, focus on something clinical or relate to clinical education. An EdD is a professional part-time doctorate in education which utilises group learning for the first two of four to five years. This might include a range of people involved in education, not necessarily all medical, offering the additional advantage of other perspectives to your work. It often provides a supported grounding in a range of methodologies and literature helping to develop ideas for a research project. While certainly not a prerequisite for all GPs who want to teach, this advanced level of educational study may be appropriate if you wish to combine general practice with an academic career. Most doctoral courses require a Masters level qualification for entry, but contact your local institution for further information. You may find that your employing institution (university, deanery or Primary Care Organisation (PCO)) contribute to fees, or you may need to apply for sponsorship elsewhere. You will also need to negotiate protected time within your timetable for study.

How do I teach?

Although being aware of possible courses and qualifications can be useful, subscription to a higher degree is something more likely to evolve *during* an established post, rather than *before* your initial teaching involvement. Here, I hope to share some of my own experience teaching undergraduates and postgraduates, to give a flavour of what a career in teaching as a GP might involve and provide some useful advice to support your teaching endeavours.

Traditionally, GPs have been less fond of didactic spoon-feeding methods of teaching delivery and are more culturally at home with learning approaches involving *co-construction* of knowledge between learner and teacher (Bruner, 1990; Piaget and Inhelder, 1969) and *facilitation* of learning or change (Rogers, 1951). The notion of the teacher as an all-powerful all-knowing provider of certainty in their specialty is, then, not a familiar sight in general practice education. Far more common is an appreciation of adult learning theory. This holds that through facilitation of discussion, either between learner and teacher or groups of learners, a learner is accessing prior experience upon which to adapt and build their knowledge, in addition to constructing and reinforcing knowledge through conversation (Bruner, 1990). This notion of teacher as 'facilitator' then moves the definition of learning from a more didactic, teacher-centred model or 'pedagogy', towards a more co-operative, learner-centred model or 'androgogy' (OED, 2010). This has important implications for the planning and preparation required for your teaching.

Firstly, it is important for you to start observing, through reflection, video or peer-feedback, how you deliver your teaching. Who does the most talking? Who asks (and even answers) the most questions? Most of us are naturally didactic, especially when anxious or pressed for time. It usually, therefore, takes time and practise (just as when practising clinical consultations) to start using open, 'Socratic' questions in order to explore where the learner is currently 'at' and allowing them to construct their subsequent path of learning. This, of course, places greater responsibility on the learner to become involved in their learning, which is not always welcome at the time. In the long-term, however, this more learner-centred approach is more likely to result in deep, retained learning (Newble and Entwistle, 1986) which (because learners better understand the processes and logic applied) is likely to be more explicitly adaptable and transferable to future situations (Eraut, 1994; Illeris, 1999; Luntley, 2007; Schon, 1983).

Secondly, by defining teaching as facilitation of learning, the involvement in teaching is broadened. Rather than exclusively 'telling' the learner what they need to know, you might design a number of heuristic activities which guide students' learning. For example, preparatory reading or presentation of a topic to the practice, internet or library tasks, in addition to direct patient experience with feedback and timely focussed one-to-one tutorials. During your initial involvement in teaching, you may be slotting into an existing teaching programme calling for less overall organisational engagement in the curriculum, or you might be asked to cover for a colleague in the practice at short notice. However, all teaching requires preparation of some sort and when first starting out, it is often these more *practical,* organisational elements which provide the most challenging, rather than worrying 'Do I know all I need to know about topic X Y and Z?'

Principles of teaching

Some useful principles about teaching, such as planning, making structure explicit and awareness of yourself as role model, might be highlighted using the example of undergraduate teaching. Teaching at this level might involve teaching on-site sessions such as generic professional skills, or small group problem-based learning, but the majority involves practice-based teaching. Practice-based teaching tends to take place at a variety of points in the curriculum in order to maximise students' exposure to patients; help them understand the spectrum of health and illness which exists; appreciate some of the contextual and community-based concerns for patients; and utilise GP's teaching skills. For example, you might teach a student practising a systems-based history for the first time with a patient, have a student based in the practice for a four-week general practice placement, or have protected teaching time for more specialised placements over a number of days, such as Child Health or Musculoskeletal Medicine. This might offer a variety of opportunities and challenges.

Planning your teaching programme requires considerable thought. The actual teaching time will be brimming with needs from patient; practice staff; student; curriculum requirements; and assessment criteria to fulfil. Planning your teaching session rarely results in delivery matching your pre-conceived vision of events. Conversely, it gives you more flexibility to choose from a variety of possible approaches to deliver a particular topic, giving you confidence to adapt a session to address students' identified learning needs as they emerge. When caught in an ad hoc situation with a student there are, in fact, many skills that you can draw on in order to confidently facilitate learning. You may not only help the student discover through Socratic questioning (open questions) what in particular it is about a topic that triggered their question, but also through role modelling, acknowledgement of uncertainty and a sense of inquiry, help students to develop crucial learning skills they will use for years to come.

For example, during a Women's Health placement, a student asks you 'Can you tell me when it is safe for a mother to start the contraceptive pill after she has given birth?' While this may be grounded in a direct patient need which the student is experiencing, and at first glance seems a purely factual question, it may also relate to a students' concerns about impending assessment, or represent wider learning for the student about, for example, attitudes towards sex, parenting, or approaches to looking up information. Using open questions in your initial exploration with the student will, therefore, help you both to identify specific areas of uncertainty for the student and focus your support. In the long-term, you may also help the student develop this process of inquiry independently, for regular use in their practice at times of 'crisis'. You might also highlight tensions between text-book management and respecting patient wishes and role model negotiation skills, or a non-judgemental attitude towards a patient which the student draws on implicitly in later professional life.

Allocating time to structuring the teaching day's topics and mode of delivery is important (*see* Box 8.3). Students are generally intelligent and motivated individuals (particularly if they are enjoying their learning). Consider then, for example, whether your time is best used to facilitate observation of a student-patient consultation with allocated reflective feedback and discussion, or delivering a factual presentation of pre-determined and accepted pathways for practice?

Box 8.3: Considering how best to deliver aspects of teaching

➤ What aspects of learning will best fit which experiences and tasks?

➤ How can I best teach this particular concern?

➤ How does this session correlate with the given curriculum or assessment?

➤ How can I vary the stimulus throughout the day to maximise students' concentration?

➤ How can I maximise the benefits of patient-based experience for the student?

➤ Which activities do I need to be directly involved in, and which can be done by the student in groups or alone?

In deciding how you are going to divide up and organise different learning activities, it is worth considering students' learning styles. Many adult-learning texts will make reference to Kolb's cycle of experiential learning (Kolb, 1984). Kolb identified four stages of learning from active involvement, reflection, incorporating relevant theory to practical application. Honey and Mumford (2006) have devised a popular questionnaire to identify in which stage of the cycle you most happily function. While it has obvious limitations in its assumptions of fixed traits, it does stimulate thought about delivery of teaching to include not only methods which fit your own preferred ways of learning, but including those of learners, which may be very different from your own. We all learn more effectively if we feel relaxed and are enjoying it (Maslow, 1943). A theorist, for example, tends to prefer to understand logic and supporting evidence prior to active involvement, whereas an activist embraces new challenge and opts straight for practical involvement. Reflectors like to be well-prepared before a session and often appear quite quiet during group discussions, but are in fact learning through observation. A pragmatist will be more motivated to learn if they understand why a session is practically relevant to them (Honey and Mumford 2006). Remember, we tend to prefer to teach using our own preferred learning style. Just as we learn and adapt a variety of consultation models to meet the needs of different patients, developing the flexibility to adapt to different ways of facilitating learning can prove a useful repertoire for the teacher.

Your relationship with the learner

Establishing an effective relationship with your learner is essential for identifying learning needs and giving feedback. Johari's window (Luft, 1984) (see adapted diagram below) can be a very useful way to visualise the ways in which you need to explore learning needs. This avoids the temptation of focussing simply upon the perceived needs of either learner or teacher, and also considers those needs which have not been expressed at all (perhaps through ignorance; focus upon 'wants' rather than needs; a desire to focus learning on areas where confidence already exists; or fear of exposing lack of knowledge). Exploring the relationship between student and teacher, Luft encourages us to think about the kinds of interaction which are required to facilitate learning (Luft, 1984). For example, learner needs assessments require a relationship of *trust* to be developed between teacher and learner. If a learner is to identify areas which are genuinely in need of attention, they need to feel that they are firstly in a comfortable environment where they can trust you to support, rather than humiliate, any inadequacies they may reveal. Secondly, it is crucial that the purpose of the session is predominantly formative (giving feedback to enhance learning), rather than summative (exam-like assessment). To a certain extent, we can probably all identify with a defence strategy to perform confidently in those areas with which we are most familiar, while deflecting or avoiding areas of unease for fear of negative effects on career progression (Lingard, 2003), but long-term, this may not represent the best approach to learning.

If as a teacher, you identify a learning need with your student, your first question might be 'Is the student aware of this need?'. Students are more likely to devote full attention to a particular topic, if they are motivated not by the teacher's awareness of a learner need, but by their own insight or 'consciousness' of their learning need or 'gap'. Once established through careful open

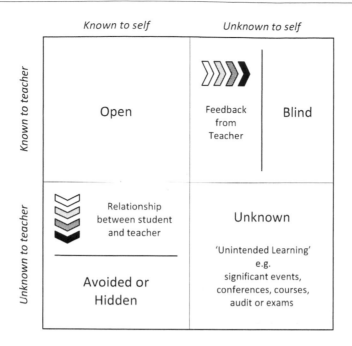

Figure 8.1: Diagram to show features of Johari's window to identify learning needs

questioning, you can plan sensitive, timely feedback to highlight areas which are, as yet, unrecognised or 'blind' to the learner. Conversely, a student might be aware of a learning need, but feel cautious about revealing this to their teacher for a number of reasons. Movement towards an open and honest exchange between learner and teacher requires the development of a trusting relationship between the two (*see* Box 8.4). Identification of learning needs unknown to both teacher and student, requires additional learning activities such as audits, video-observation or attending conferences. For further discussion of learning needs, *see* Chapter 7: Professional development.

The importance of the student-teacher relationship is particularly important for providing feedback. General practice, certainly at an undergraduate level, is often one of the few places where a student can build a meaningful relationship with one teacher over a period of time enabling trust and formative comments to be made. Similar to clinical consultations, often the most effective way to establish what level to pitch comments is to allow the learner to speak first. The vast majority of students have insight and allowing them to share their concerns first will often help them be more receptive to any additional comments you make. Most GPs are familiar with Pendleton's model of giving feedback which involves the learner, then tutor saying what went well, followed by the learner, then tutor saying what could

---

Box 8.4: How you can maximise the development of a trusting relationship between teacher and learner in general practice

➤ Punctuality on both parts
➤ Arrange in advance how patient appointments will be aligned with teaching delivery to balance teaching and service commitments.
➤ Plan how you will start the session, in order to give students a sense of commitment from you – even the briefest of outlines about the structure can make learners feel that the teaching has been specifically thought out with their learning in mind.
➤ Provide space (however brief) for summarising and exchanging feedback at regular intervals.
➤ Begin by briefly setting ground rules and boundaries (generated from both parties) and clarifying what individuals are hoping to get out of the teaching. Return to these regularly, for a sense of completion, focus and achievement.
➤ Make sure other staff in the practice is aware that the teaching is happening. It is useful to ask receptionists to respect teaching time as they would a consultation, avoiding interruptions wherever possible. Colleagues may make additional efforts to support sessions by popping in if a relevant patient is happy to be involved, or providing a newly acquired piece of relevant literature.
➤ Be honest, if you can, as this will generally reciprocate respect and honesty from the students.

---

be improved with possible suggestions (Pendleton *et al*, 1984). The principle of this process is to provide balanced feedback. We all tend to criticise ourselves before thinking of positive comments, when in fact, we may need at least five positive comments to one negative to feel we have received 'balanced feedback' (Gottman, 1994). A more outcome-based way to facilitate feedback can be the Calgary–Cambridge model (Silverman, Draper and Kurtz, 1997), which asks the learner what they were aiming to achieve, what they would like specific help with, what went well, what could be improved with alternative strategies and then providing an opportunity for role-play or rehearsal of alternatives.

How do I involve patients?

Balancing clinical and teaching needs during a session can be a challenging business. As in the consultation, you as a 'doctor-teacher' have an agenda for curriculum delivery, in addition to learner-identified needs. You will also have to manage the patient-agendas which willing volunteers bring to the session, while also identifying and addressing areas of particular benefit to the student. Balancing student and patient agendas is an important art as there is an element of altruism on the part of the patient in consenting to participate in this educational endeavour. Doubtless, there will be reciprocal benefits for the patient (*see* Boxes 8.5 and 8.6). Patients, for example, are often very sensitive to the subtle changes in power-relationship between doctor and student, and so feel much freer to ask for explanations about their concerns. They may also be interested to hear what you, as teacher, add to the discussions. You may either choose to focus upon the detail of their particular experience, or expand the discussions to more generalisable areas from within the consultation. Through indirectly sharing your expertise and knowledge with patients, they often experience a sense of positivity towards their condition or predicament.

Box 8.5: Advantages to sharing student-teacher discussions with patients

➤ Sense of relief for the patient at generalisability of their concern or experience.

➤ Sense of empowerment for the patient at gaining a better understanding of the medical knowledge surrounding their own experience.

➤ Patients have greater control to determine which confidential aspects of their story they are happy to share in this context.

➤ Patients are often able to contribute, supplement and develop relevant discussions.

➤ Discussions and feedback are likely to be more meaningful for the student if they are happening at the time.

Box 8.6: Disadvantages to sharing student-teacher discussions with the patient

➤ It is important to judge the readiness of both audiences (student and patient) to receive certain elements of information. Once absorbed in teaching, it is easy to forget that the patient or relatives are listening. Similarly, a patient may have agreed to participate in teaching, but become uncomfortable if the session starts to expose an unexpected topic or area.

➤ If not made explicit beforehand, extending discussions beyond a particular circumstance can cause anxiety for the patient about potential side-effects, complications or prognosis.

➤ Whereas it is easy to give positive feedback in front of patients, criticism can be embarrassing for the student to receive and also challenge patients' preconceptions of medical expertise. Patients can, however, be a very valuable asset to the delivery of feedback to students about aspects of their consulting approach.

How can I support students moving towards professional practice?

Learners usually want to succeed. Like patients, learners often seek certainty in their quest to achieve the required outcomes within their training. Although uncomfortable, it is often this sense of uncertainty which motivates learning. The privilege of the teacher in primary care is an opportunity to facilitate learning beyond the standard protocols and practice guidelines which will undoubtedly change with time. GPs can help support students in their development as medical professionals, using many of the skills which they are familiar using with patients. The principle of valuing the individual, the 'self' (Balint, 1957), can help nurture a genuine commitment to the personal qualities required of the professional, rather than those simply desired by external regulatory authorities.

Students are often torn between prioritising their own empathetic and intuitive responses to observations of patients' perspectives and experience, with the perceived need to impose a disease-orientated model upon the situation. They are searching for role models of 'sound judgement' to inform their practice and are often balancing the capacity to act with courage, in spite of fears, risks and uncertainties, with the humility to recognise their existing weaknesses and strengths (bacp, 2010). This humility is often mixed with a desire not to offend the boundaries of power and hierarchy within medical training, which assume that experience and seniority make a doctor's practice more likely to be correct, together with the expected dual roles of teachers as professional colleague and summative assessor.

This relation of power means that you, as teacher, have the responsibility to set the tone of conversation between teacher and student. You have the choice to communicate with this student as a professional colleague, with all the increased challenges and responsibilities this brings to the student, or you choose a more traditional adoption of the child-adult model. As with consulting styles, your repertoire choice may vary according to the patient situation and needs, student engagement and required tasks within the teaching session. These assumed hierarchical relations of power within training, mean that a student is unlikely to enquire or challenge an element of practice which they have observed, unless given the opportunity to do so, within an open and respectful environment. Your decision-making, for example, may be influenced by multiple factors, all of which you will not have time to explain (*see* Box 8.7). However, when being observed, asking an open question between patient appointments may briefly allow you to address, and make explicit, an area of influence upon your practice, enriching both your own awareness and the learning of the student.

Box 8.7: Possible factors influencing our practice which are often implicit, but useful to consider sharing or making explicit in discussions about decision-making and management with students

➤ Priorities of the particular patient.
➤ Historical demands (wants) or needs of this patient, their family or relatives.
➤ PCO rationing directorates.
➤ Policy documents (e.g. NICE guidelines, prescribing recommendations, GMC guidance, medical school teaching material).
➤ Concerns about the measurement of quality as an outcome of the consultation e.g. scores for the quality and outcomes framework (QOF), personal judgements about our professional conduct by colleagues receiving referrals, patient survey reports, patient complaints, relationship with colleagues within the practice).
➤ GP teacher's own health and well-being on that particular day.
➤ Time-constraints affecting decisions to tackle or defer particular issues in that consultation.

During these discussions, students are often able to make a reciprocal contribution to the practice workings, by offering their own perspectives on consultations and management plans. Whereas an experienced GPs vision or perspective of the consultation has been coloured by the consideration of various demands or lenses, students may be able to offer a highly sensitive, and often more patient-centred interpretation of the consultation. Rather than dismissing this, often more emotionally colourful, narrative of events, consider stopping and thinking about how this perspective could provide additional ways of approaching a particular issue or context. Our habitual response within medicine is often to assume that the disease-orientated model is the most effective and efficient way of understanding a consultation. Given space, other paradigms suggested by students can, however, provide an additional richness with potential benefits for patient care and practitioner well-being. Conversely, a student may be so intent on mastering the disease-orientated framework that they need support learning to successfully integrate this into a particular patient context, developing the flexibility to engage an empathetic position within their practice.

Making space for these dialogues, does not necessarily take lengthy periods of time. It is, however, important to structure time within the sessions, in order to provide a meaningful reflective dimension to the students' learning experience. A large part of learning is about making sense or meaning of our experience. We do this by trying to fit accepted or desirable discourses (or a particular way of understanding) with our own interpretations. Allowing students to look at a complex clinical consultation from a number of different perspectives may help broaden an awareness of practice which is determined not only by one, but many voices – often in tension with each other. Understanding how you, as a role model, begin to firstly understand then prioritise these demands has many benefits. Firstly, students can gain an appreciation of the diversity of good practice within Medicine, shifting from the simplistic conception that there exists a specific standard and accepted mode of practice to be replicated in exams, towards a more complex appreciation of a valuable repertoire of approaches to practice which suit multiple patient and practice contexts. Secondly, it can help students begin to understand when to tolerate and how to recognise and address uncertainty within their own professional experience. Thirdly, in articulating such discussions for students, our own reflective learning can in fact benefit subsequent practice.

Teaching safely

Just as we have discussed students acknowledging and learning to manage uncertainty within their experience of the consultation, as teachers we also need to manage the uncertainty and sometimes, challenging feelings of inviting a student into our professional world. Particularly, if you are beginning to maximise a students' learning opportunities by asking them to consult, there is an element of risk involved. You can, however, make this risk feel more comfortable, in a number of ways. The approach you take to this will depend heavily upon the experience of the students and curricular aims and constraints. Is this, for example, a four-week placement with your practice, two days focussed upon a certain topic, or a postgraduate placement lasting several months? It will also depend, to an extent, upon how many students you are responsible for teaching. Co-ordinating groups in pairs, alternating the roles of observer (and feedback-giver) with practitioner, can be useful particularly at undergraduate level.

Get to know your student through discussion and observation in practice. This way, you can develop rapport and trust, in addition to understanding their strengths and weaknesses. You may then choose to facilitate the shift in clinical responsibility in small stages. For example, you may begin by arranging for the student to observe your own consultations, offering regular opportunities for discussion. Next, try swapping seats at points in the consultation to allow the student consulting experience, in the relatively safe context of your observation. This can work well if negotiated beforehand but prove challenging, even threatening, for an unsuspecting student grappling to develop their knowledge and consulting style. Make sure you arrange the seating so that a familiar patient is not tempted to address you, rather than the student. Next, perhaps arrange (where space allows) for students to consult in a neighbouring room. You can then decide how you will arrange appointments in order to allow periods for feedback and discussion, in addition to making sure that patients' expressed needs have been acknowledged or addressed.

Try, if you can, to negotiate appointment times, within the practice service demands, to allow space at regular intervals for discussion. No teacher will be able to fully prioritise their student's needs while filling with anxiety about a packed waiting room and weighty dose of impending home visits and paperwork. You might, for example, consult for one hour from 08.00, then prepare to welcome a student and restart at 10.00 with the student, planning either a couple of catch up breaks mid-surgery or arrange slightly longer appointment times. You will always need to consider the purpose of the teaching session when arranging appointment times, in addition to balancing the service demands of the practice. Generally, teaching will be paid to reflect the amount of protected teaching time (as opposed to concurrent service work) required. Whereas undergraduates may need continued support during a clinical session, at postgraduate level, with time, you may wish to negotiate less regular interruption as learners become more confident at problem-solving and prioritising, building towards independent practice. You still, however, need to protect regular allocated time during the week as planned space for discussion.

You will need to consider how the existing infrastructure, supporting the safety of individuals within your practice, can be extended to students. Preparing a 'student pack' with relevant information for them to read or discuss may be helpful as preparatory material and give them a sense of belonging to the practice environment. It is also advisable to ring your insurance provider, just to confirm current guidance on teaching in your practice. Students should also hold a suitable policy with an insurer, but check with the responsible medical school or deanery. If you are worried or have concerns about a student which you wish to discuss, you should always be able to approach the institution supporting your teaching for advice. Establishing an open and trusting relationship with your student, however, will anticipate and support you through most presenting difficulties. Try and establish a culture of honesty, where you too acknowledge that mistakes happen and offer collaborative solutions, wherever possible.

Conclusion

Just as we refine and improve our consultations through years of experience, reflection and openness to new knowledge and practices, so too our teaching changes and evolves with time. Many of the initial hurdles involve the more pragmatic considerations about organisation and negotiations within the practice. Once established, however, clinical practice, teacher, patient and student can flourish given the opportunity. Teaching, as with being a GP, is an enormous privilege whether involved in practice-based delivery, organisation and management, research or all three elements. With positive motives and enthusiasm, it can prove incredibly rewarding and also help to develop and refine our professional selves, with many clinical, educational and personal rewards.

Some relevant qualifications in medical education

These are a selection of courses and institutions available at the time of publication. Although we have tried to search for all available courses and institutions, this may not be a comprehensive list and course availability and institutions may, of course, change over time.

Institutions offering intercalated BSc (iBSc) level courses

Barts and the London School of Medicine and Dentistry – iBSc in Medical Education
Leeds Institute of Medical Education – iBSc in Medical Education

Institutions offering Masters level courses

Most of these institutions offer Masters level qualifications. Many of these courses offer interim qualifications of a certificate (after one year of study) or diploma (after two years of study). Completion of a Masters level qualification also usually includes a dissertation. Most are part-time and would be completed concurrent with your existing working role. Dundee, however, does offer an additional 'intensive' option to complete a Masters course full-time over one year, in addition to their part-time distance learning route.

➤ Anglia Ruskin University – MSc in Medical and Healthcare Education
➤ University of Sussex – Brighton – MA Education Studies
➤ Bristol – MMedSci MSc in Teaching and Learning for Health Professionals
➤ University of Bedfordshire – MA Medical Education
➤ University of Belfast – MMedSc Clinical Education
➤ University of Cardiff – MSc Medical Education
➤ University of Dundee – MMEd Medical Education (Full time or distance learning)
➤ University of Durham – MSc Medical Education
➤ University of East Anglia (UEA) – M Clin Ed Clinical Education
➤ University of Essex – MSc in Medical and Clinical Education
➤ Glasgow – MSC (MedSci) Health-Professions Education
➤ Institute of Education & London Deanery – MA Clinical Education
➤ Kings College London – MA Education and Professional Studies
➤ Keele – MA Medical Education
➤ Leeds University – MEd in Clinical Education or MSc in Educational Research Methods
➤ Newcastle – M Clin Ed Master of Clinical Education, MA Education Research
➤ Nottingham – MMedSci Medical Education Masters
➤ UCL – M Clin Ed in Clinical Education, or MSc (with Royal College of Physicians) Medical Education
➤ University of Westminster & London Deanery – Postgraduate Certificate for Teachers in Primary Care (Teaching the Teachers or TTT)
➤ Sheffield – MMedSci, MA Educational Research
➤ Warwick – MMedEd in Medical Education
➤ Peninsula Medical School (PMS) – M Clin Ed in Clinical Education

Institutions offering Professional Doctorates in Education

These are usually four to five years in length part-time (i.e. concurrent with your usual working role), with a maximum completion time of seven to eight years. You will usually be awarded a doctorate in education (EdD or DEd). Most doctorates (unless otherwise stated) are open to anyone involved in education (offering an excellent learning resource), but you can develop your own focus relevant to your professional context.

➤ Institute of Education, University of London
➤ University of Belfast
➤ University of Keele
➤ University of Dundee
➤ University of Huddersfield
➤ University of Hertfordshire
➤ University of Sussex (Brighton)
➤ University of Bristol
➤ University of Cardiff
➤ University of Newcastle
➤ University of East Anglia
➤ University of Glasgow (Health-Professions Education)
➤ University of Sheffield (EdD in Higher Education)

Relevant organisations and what they do

Association for the Study of Medical Education (ASME) – arrange various events and conferences including an annual conference in association with the Researching Medical Learning and Practice Network (based at the Institute of Education) called 'Researching Medical Education'. They also publish various documents and the journal *Medical Education*. www.asme.org.uk

The Association for Medical Education in Europe (AMEE) has a more international flavour. They publish a number of documents and the journal *Medical Teacher*. www.amee.org

Academy of Medical Educators – is a relatively new body seeking to provide a college equivalent organisation to support and perhaps in the future regulate medical educators' development. They have produced some recommendations on professional standards for use in curricula. www.medicaleducators.org

Society of Academic Primary Care (SAPC) – arrange conferences and publish the journal of *Primary Healthcare Research and Development* below. They are an international organisation and offer support to GPs involved in research and education. www.sapc.ac.uk

The Higher Education Academy (HEA) offers a range of support for members in addition to recognition for teaching activity by submission of a written report, which may be useful for job applications and career development. www.heacademy.ac.uk

The Postgraduate Medical Education and Training Board (PMETB) was responsible for regulating postgraduate training. They merged in April 2010 with the GMC who are now responsible for the regulation of all stages of medical education and training. www.pmetb.org.uk

The Royal College of General Practice (RCGP) and your local deanery may also offer courses and communications, particularly around postgraduate education. www.rcgp.org.uk and www.gprecruitment.org.uk/deaneries.htm

National Association of Primary Care Educators is an inter-disciplinary organisation for GP tutors and programme directors. They are associated with the *Journal of Education for Primary Care*. www.napce.net

Publications of interest

➤ *Medical Education*
➤ *Medical Teacher*
➤ *Journal of Education for Primary Care ('the green journal')*
➤ *Primary Healthcare Research and Development*
➤ *British Journal of General Practice*

References

BACP. *BACP: ethical framework*; 2010. [Online]. Available at: www.bacp.co.uk/ethical_framework/personal.php (accessed 24 January 2010).

Balint M. *The Doctor, His Patient and the Illness*. London: Pitman Medical Publishing Co; 1957.

BMA. *Teacher Education in the Medical Profession*. London: BMA; 2006.

Bruner J. *Acts of Meaning*. Cambridge, MA: Harvard University Press; 1990.

Eraut M. *Developing Professional Knowledge and Competence*. London: The Falmer Press; 1994.

GMC. *Tomorrow's Doctors*; 2009. [Online]. Available at: www.gmc-uk.org/education/documents/GMC_TD_2009.pdf (accessed 28 September 2009).

Gottman M. *What Predicts Divorce: The Relationship Between Marital Processes and Marital Outcomes*. New Jersey: Lawrence Erlbaum Associates; 1994.

Honey P, Mumford A. *Learning Styles Helper's Guide*. Maidenhead: Peter Honey Publications; 2006.

Illeris K. *How We Learn: Learning and non-learning in school and beyond*. London: Routledge; 1999.

Kolb DA. *Experiential Learning: Experience as the source for learning and development*. Englewood Cliffs, NJ: Prentice-Hall; 1984.

Lingard L, Garwood K, Schryer CF, et al. A certain art of uncertainty: case presentation and the development of professional identity. *Social Science and Medicine*. 2003; **56**: 603–616.

Luft J. Group processes: an introduction to group dynamics. *Proceedings of the Western Training Laboratory in Group Development* (pp. 60–78). Palo Alto, CA: Mayfield Publishing; 1984.

Luntley M. Care, sensibility and judgement. In: Drummond JS, Standish P (eds). *The Philosophy of Nurse Education*. Basingstoke: Palgrave Macmillan; 2007, pp. 77–90.

Maslow A. A theory of human motivation. *Psychological Review.* 1943; **5**: 370–396.

Newble DI, Entwistle NJ. Learning styles and approaches: implications for medical education. *Medical Education.* 1986; **20**: 162–175.

OED. *Oxford English Dictionary;* 2010. [Online]. Available at: www.askoxford. com/concise_oed/doctor?view=uk (accessed 21 April 2010).

Pendleton D, Schofield T, Tate P, *et al. The Consultation: An Approach to Learning and Teaching*. Oxford: Oxford University Press; 1984.

Piaget J, Inhelder B. *The Psychology of the Child*. London: Routledge and Kegan Paul; 1969.

Rogers C. *Client-centered Therapy: Its current practice, implications and theory*. Boston: Houghton Mifflin; 1951.

Schon DA. *The Reflective Practitioner: How professionals think in action*. London: Arena, Ashgate Publishing Ltd; 1983.

Silverman JD, Draper J, Kurtz SM. The Calgary–Cambridge approach in communication skills teaching 2: The SET-GO method of descriptive feedback. *Education in General Practice.* 1997; **8**: 16–23.

Career profile:

Ann Griffin

When did you qualify?

I qualified from King's College London School of Medicine in 1985.

What is your job?

I work as a Senior Clinical Lecturer in Medical Education in the Division of Medical Education at UCL Medical School and am the sub-Dean for Quality. I also work as a Sessional GP in North London.

Why and how did you choose General Practice and then teaching?

I think it is fair to say that I fell into both general practice and teaching, I don't remember making a particularly active choice about either. When I qualified, I wanted to become a hospital physician and did a series of very interesting posts in general medicine, cardiology, haematology, neurology, endocrinology and neuro-otology but two things always bothered me – the prospect of endless nights spent on-call and further medical exams. Thinking that general practice sounded better, I did obstetrics and gynaecology, A&E, care of the older person and paediatrics before getting a post as a GP registrar. Once qualified as a GP, I worked as a locum and then in salaried posts. One of the surgeries that employed me, in fact, the place where I still work, asked me if I'd like to teach medical students. I said yes thinking it would make a nice change to seeing patients full time. That, little known to me at the time, was the beginning of my new career. From teaching in my practice, I took up an academic post in the Division of Population Sciences at UCL. Despite my earlier reluctance to take more examinations, joining the department made me think more constructively about gaining higher qualifications. I started with my MRCGP, then went on to a Masters in Medical Education and am now in the last stages of a professional doctorate in education.

What do you do?

I left primary care as my academic base just recently to join the Division of Medical Education, as it was clear my interests in teaching and learning were no longer constrained by my clinical specialty. So, now I help healthcare professionals develop as educators, run postgraduate courses with colleagues, support the quality assurance of the undergraduate curriculum and research into various aspects of medical education…and see patients.

What is the most rewarding aspect of your job?

I think the people I work with: colleagues in particular. I also like the variety, stimulation and the creativity of working within an academic environment.

What is the most challenging or frustrating thing about your job?

There is always so much you could get involved in, which is great, but you have to be realistic. Working as a portfolio GP means you need to be a good multi-tasker and sometimes you just have to say no.

If you could change one thing about your career what would it be?

Nothing. My career path may be perceived as a bit tortuous but I consider the opportunity to have all these experiences as being a great privilege.

What do you wish you knew then that you know now?

I wish I had known that there was a job, or combinations of roles, that would tick all the boxes: worthwhile, satisfying, creative, flexible, challenging etc. No-one said. So my advice, go ask, experiment and enjoy – it's never too late.

Reflective piece: 'Family education'

Pauline Bryant

With current maternity leave and rights, women tend to get paid maternity leave to enjoy their new baby. This is great, but it can have a downside. Return to work is a very common topic of conversation among mothers. Many women worry about whether they will cope and are concerned that their memory and concentration have deteriorated after the birth of their child. I'm not sure if this is a clinical fact, but I would certainly think it could be related to sleep deprivation. While away from work, it seems common for women to worry that they have deskilled, but it is important to separate competence from confidence. It is unlikely that clinical skills will have decayed too much in six or even twelve months.

As a GP, I always felt very fortunate that the things I had learned as a parent gave me a new 'skill set' directly relevant and useful for my job. This was not the case for friends with other careers. I loved being at home on maternity leave but realised that, as the baby grew, so did the cleaning, tidying and washing! This I did not enjoy. I found a nursery that I was happy with, and a cleaner, and returned to work part time.

I had been teaching before the maternity leave and now found that teaching helped me to catch up more quickly. I would highly recommend teaching as a way to keep up to date as it encourages you to look up and discuss latest guidelines. It is great for appraisal and revalidation too. I was also registered on a distance learning part-time Masters in Medical education course and this was possible to do from home and flexible enough to accommodate career breaks – it took seven years but was worth it. It was good to have an academic goal.

Ten years on and four children later, my reflections would be that I have managed to combine a career in medicine and motherhood that I am very happy with. I was always interested in academic general practice and teaching in particular. I found that this fitted very well with having a family. Teaching and medical school work hours can be more flexible than general practice, so sports days and assemblies can be attended if you are prepared to work in the evenings. Although, financially, teaching may not be as well-paid as clinical practice, quality of life may be better.

Having taken lengthy maternity leave, and worked part-time, I have not climbed the academic career ladder quickly. But, I have had time to see my family and really enjoyed the last ten years which have whizzed by. I remain driven but I am also able to take time to reflect on what is really important in life. The children are no longer babies but the career doors are all still open. I am ready for the next challenge. I am about to start an Educational Doctorate.

CHAPTER 9

International primary care

Luisa Pettigrew and Iona Heath

Introduction

Have you ever wondered what it would be like to work in another country? How other primary healthcare systems work? What GP training is like outside the UK? Wanted to have a better understanding of the cultural differences you encounter in your day-to-day practice? Felt that you wanted to contribute to improve global health? Felt that you needed a new challenge? If so, perhaps an experience in international primary care may give you the answer you are looking for.

The diversity of general practice education, clinical care, primary care systems, health beliefs, cultures, pathology and health outcomes across the world are as immense as the benefits of learning about them. The kind of overseas experiences that exist are also varied; some are immediately recognisable as general practice, whereas others draw on the wider sense of primary care for which an even greater diversity of skills are required. Also, bear in mind that not all international experiences mean that you need to commit to a long period overseas or even have to leave the UK!

We hope that this chapter will help you to explore some of these opportunities.

Why do it?

Stepping out of work in the UK to undertake an international experience can broaden your horizons, giving you a fresh perspective of what it means to be a General Practitioner. Through working overseas and learning about international health issues you will acquire new skills, many of which are applicable and beneficial to the NHS. These can include clinical, teaching, management, leadership, cultural and organisational skills (*see* Figure 9.1). New experiences can also re-invigorate you, giving you a heightened sense of vocation which will propel you through your career. Furthermore, travelling with your career will bring you new friendships, which will foster personal

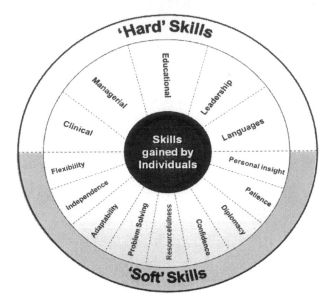

Figure 9.1: Skills gained by individual health workers. Tribal Newchurch adapted from Lord Darzi's Next Stage Review, 2009 (DH, 2010a)

and professional development. You may even learn a new language! As a result of your international experience, the NHS will have a more skilled and motivated workforce (Banatvala, 1997a; Banatvala, 1997b; Crawford, 2009; Crisp, 2007; Crisp, 2010; DH, 2005; DH, 2010a; Holden, 1998; Koehn, 2006; Machin, 2008; Tan, 2005).

Working overseas helps to develop a better understanding of the political and socio-economic factors which affect health, and greater insight to alternative healthcare initiatives. The growth of international partnerships may also lead to a more cohesive and collaborative approach to improving global health. In addition, the quality of healthcare and medical education can improve at an international level through the increased dialogue among medical organisations (Davis, 1998; Grol, 2007; Legido-Quigley, 2008). In fact, what we know as general practice today has inevitably been influenced along the way by primary care overseas (Horder, 1990; Johnstone, 1995).

Global Health versus International Health

The terms 'Global Health' and 'International Health' are being increasingly used, and may be assumed to mean the same thing. However, the UK's Department of Health differentiates them:

'Global Health' is increasingly used to describe health issues that are affected by a complex array of direct and indirect global forces, and solving problems often requires multilateral co-operation across a range of sectors.

'International Health' has traditionally been more about contrasts between health practices, policies and systems in different countries. (DH, 2009)

When should I go?

As a student

Whilst at medical school, most students will have had an opportunity to experience working in another country during the elective period. As a student, you may also have had overseas contact through 'Medsin', the UK affiliation of the International Federation of Medical Students' Associations (IFMSA). In addition, a few UK Medical Schools now offer an intercalated BSc in International or Global Health, and some, an optional, shorter, student-selected component or module within the undergraduate medical curriculum.

As a trainee

As discussed in Chapter 2: General practice specialty training, since the introduction of Modernising Medical Careers, once you finish medical school you go straight into your foundation years and normally progress immediately through to GP training. A very limited number of foundation year four-month-long international health posts emerged in recent years, yet overall, the flexibility to choose to take time out during training seems to have become a little more rigid. However, the independent inquiry into Modernising Medical Careers, 'Aspiring to Excellence' recommended that Time Out of Programme should be,

'positively facilitated and encouraged, given that such out of programme activity enriches the skill base and professional life of doctors, as well as promoting research and development, and the global health agenda'

Tooke, 2008

The Gold Guide, which is the reference document that provides guidance to UK postgraduate deans on the arrangements for specialty training, clarifies that there are four different kinds of Time Out of Programme (OOP) (DH, 2010).

➤ Time out of programme for approved clinical training (OOPT)
➤ Time out of programme for research (OOPR)
➤ Time out of programme for clinical experience (OOPE)
➤ Time out of programme for career breaks (OOPC)

All types of time OOP must be approved by your postgraduate dean. However OOPT and OOPR must also be prospectively approved by the GMC, if it is to count towards the award of a certificate of completion of training (CCT). OOPE does not require GMC approval as such an experience is not a requirement of the curriculum. OOPC does not require approval beyond the deanery either.

For GP trainees, most opportunities to work overseas will fall under the OOPE category, and will usually only be granted between ST2 and ST3. In some cases, it may be possible to gain partial recognition of the overseas experience for it to count towards your CCT. For example, of a twelve-month overseas placement, six months may be recognised as training. The decision as to whether the overseas experience will count towards training is based on the individual application and, if accepted, you will be expected to submit regular assessments of progress (e.g. via e-Portfolio) and a final report. OOPE and OOPT will normally be for one year in total, however, in exceptional cases this may be extended to two years.

The Gold Guide recommends the minimum notice to prepare time OOP is 3 months, however, in practice you will probably need at least 6–12 months. Therefore the earlier you apply, the greater the chances are of you being able to successfully organise time OOP.

For more details on organising time OOP please refer to the Gold Guide and a helpful article entitled 'Time out' published in BMJ Careers (Spry, 2008). The BMA's International Department has also developed a comprehensive guidance document for doctors entitled, 'Broadening your horizons: a guide to taking time out to work and train in developing countries' (BMA, 2009a).

As a qualified GP

As has been previously discussed in this book, once you qualify, you may be working as a locum GP, salaried GP, GP partner, an academic GP or even a combination of these. As a locum, you have the freedom to choose when to work, therefore, such work may provide the flexibility and opportunity to raise funds to go overseas. As a salaried GP, some practices may be willing to consider unpaid leave. In some cases, your primary care organisation may support your practice to enable you to take extended study leave. Similarly, as an academic GP, it will depend upon the discretion of your employer although there may be opportunities to incorporate international research into your work (*see* below). Some GP partnerships have a sabbatical period contracted into the partnership agreement. Sabbaticals can work well if they have been carefully agreed, including arrangements on how your clinical work will be covered, how it will affect your partnership drawings and how decisions will be made in your absence.

You should also bear in mind that there are many exciting and enlightening international experiences that can take place within a week or two of leave, such as attending an international primary care conference, or being an expedition medic. You can even have an international experience without leaving the UK, for example, by hosting a visiting exchange doctor in your practice or through becoming involved with UK refugee and asylum seeker support organisations locally.

As a retired GP

Finally, retirement may also offer the time to fulfil lifelong ambitions of international work. Most overseas clinical work will require you to have a GMC licence to practise, however with the enormous breadth of skills and experience you will have, there are also numerous opportunities to undertake non-clinical work such as teaching, management or even medical journalism.

Considerations

Appraisal and revalidation

The implications of revalidation for doctors working overseas are not yet completely clear but it seems that all the relevant organisations are committed to ensuring that the revalidation system does not discourage UK doctors from working overseas.

If you are only abroad for a limited period of time and will be in the UK at the time of revalidation, the RCGP is suggesting two routes. You can collect supporting information and submit a standard revalidation portfolio to your responsible officer. For a standard revalidation portfolio, the RCGP will expect within a 5 year period at least three annual appraisals done within the NHS system and three years' worth of learning credits (50 credits per year). In addition, you will need to have done at least 200 clinical half-day sessions as a GP in the UK in the 5 years of the revalidation cycle. You may wish to organise locum work in the UK in order to meet this requirement.

If this is not possible, then you should submit what supporting evidence you can and your responsible officer will consider it as an exceptional portfolio. The responsible officer, perhaps after consulting the RCGP, will reach a view and make a recommendation to the GMC where the final decision will be made. You may be revalidated for a shorter period than five years.

However, if you are abroad when your revalidation is due, you may not be able to apply to be revalidated. Although your licence will be suspended you will be in 'good standing' and should be able to continue to work overseas. When you return, the GMC will apply a process to re-issue your licence. This may require future revalidation in less than the usual five years. Employers are likely to also want to know that you are fit to practise in the UK, and this may require you to update appropriately. If you have been working as a GP in a developed country, you may only need to refresh on guidelines, commissioning and NHS systems. If, however, you have been working in a developing country for many years, you may also need to refresh your knowledge on chronic disease management etc.

Whichever of these three scenarios you think will apply to you, the important thing is to collect what revalidation supporting information you can. You should maintain a portfolio which documents your learning needs, personal development plans and learning activities.

More details will become available as revalidation gets underway and information will be made available by both the GMC (www.gmc-uk.org) and the RCGP (www.rcgp.org.uk).

Performer's List

To work as a GP in the UK, in addition to GMC registration, you are required to be listed on the local Performers' List. Currently, you may be removed from a Performers' List if you cannot demonstrate that you have performed any primary medical services within that list's area during the preceding 12 months. You will also find it difficult to be accepted onto a Performers' List after more than two years out of UK general practice. Therefore, at present, the situation is considerably less than ideal, and the BMA advise that GPs working overseas return at least once within a twelve-month period to do locum work, thus enabling continuation on the Performer's List for a further twelve-month period. Practices can vary slightly across the UK. Your Local Medical Committee (LMC) should be able to offer further guidance on how to remain on your local Performer's List. Being on a Performer's List is also important as they provide your appraiser and once revalidation is underway they will appoint your responsible officer. However, at the time of writing, with current NHS proposals in England, this is subject to change!

Pension

If you are working overseas, your pension contributions will normally stop when you cease to be paid by the NHS and will resume on your return. Also, if you leave your current pension scheme, on return, you may have to enter under a new scheme. Recent regulations have allowed employees to choose to pay contributions for the first 6 months, with their employer continuing to pay their part. Thereafter, you can pay both your own and the employer's contribution for up to a further 18 months. As there are numerous variables, dependant on what kind of employment contract you have, and how long you will be away for, it is advisable that you seek further information and guidance from the NHS Pension Scheme (www.nhsbsa.nhs.uk) and the BMA (www.bma.org.uk).

Health, safety and medical indemnity

Before you leave, make sure you have all your vaccines up-to-date and take anti-malarial medication, if necessary. Find out if you are likely to be exposed to HIV infection, and consider discussing, with the local infectious diseases department, if post exposure prophylaxis (PEP) would be appropriate. Remember also, that road traffic accidents are one of the most common causes of death for people travelling or working overseas. Therefore avoid situations that may put you at risk and ensure you have the appropriate travel insurance. If you are going to undertake clinical work, ensure you have medical indemnity and licence to practise, if required. It is worth noting that you may find it harder to secure indemnity cover if there is a possibility that an USA or Canadian citizen may take action against you in their own country. Understandably, it may also be harder to find travel insurance if you chose to visit an unstable country.

Culture shock

One of the challenges you may face, is that of the need to adapt to a new culture. You may encounter very different ways of working, dealing with others and health beliefs. Therefore, research the country you plan to visit. Many countries which you may choose to visit will be poorer, without the infrastructure and resources that the UK is fortunate to have. Therefore, be prepared to feel frustrated, sad and even angry at times. In addition in most countries, although you may find some people who speak English, understandably, most of the work will need to be done through interpreters, who may not be medically trained. In view of this, a medical language course may prove a wise investment. Finally, if you choose to work in a region of war or conflict, going with a recognised agency that offers you appropriate security training and training on international humanitarian laws and practice is strongly advisable. Also, be aware of the potential psychological impact that working in this setting may have on you. Prepare yourself, and ensure you know how to access help and support when you need it.

Ethical considerations

Through undertaking work overseas you will inevitably have an impact in some shape or form. It is, therefore, imperative that you consider carefully exactly what impact you expect to have. When considering undertaking development or relief work with an organisation, be it governmental or non-governmental, it is important to bear in mind that projects which are locally led and foster long-term partnerships increase the likelihood of the results being longer lasting, sustainable and positive for all parties (Crisp, 2010).

As highlighted by the World Health Organization 2006 report and Global Workforce Alliance, there is a global shortage of 4.2 million health professionals, which is particularly felt in developing countries due to the recognised 'brain-drain' and the lack of training opportunities (WHO, 2006). Initiatives through which local communities are empowered to be able to provide their own healthcare are a step towards reversing this shortage.

You may also find yourself in situations where you are asked to undertake clinical work that you would not normally do in the UK. You will need to carefully reflect on the pros and cons and potential consequences of doing so, before venturing forth. The Centre for International Health and Development at University College London published the, 'Guide to Global Health Electives' (Pollit, 2009) which, although an elective pack aimed at undergraduates, offers very useful advice for anyone planning to work in a developing country. The BMA has also published relevant guidance in its document 'Ethics and medical electives in resource-poor countries: a toolkit' (BMA, 2009b).

Finally, although inevitably you will have to travel to your destination, think about your carbon footprint and consider ways to keep this at a minimum.

So, what can I actually do?

The kind of work or experience you undertake may include clinical service, health promotion, health prevention, research, teaching or management. It could also involve public health or health policy. It could be a short observational placement, exchange, expedition or international conference. Therefore before rushing into anything ask yourself:

➤ What do I want to do?
➤ What can I offer?

➤ What do I expect to get out of it?
➤ What are the needs and expectations of where I want to go to?
➤ How long can I go for?
➤ What happens when I come back?

Once you have considered this, below you will find an introduction to examples of international experiences that you may be able to combine with a career in general practice. Following this, on page 161, you will find a list outlining some of the organisations involved in international primary care which may help facilitate such an experience.

Working in a developing country

Relief versus Development

Relief work is usually short-term and related to manmade or natural disasters. It can also be called humanitarian work. However due to the long-lasting impact of many disasters, relief work is often also integrated with development work. Development work focuses on making sustainable changes to a community through local participation, education and a holistic approach. Most relief and development work is undertaken in low or middle income countries, otherwise often referred to as developing countries.

There is a chasm of inequalities of health and healthcare provision across the world (WHO, 2010). As you can imagine, the reason for this is multifactorial and, as a result, numerous non-governmental organisations (NGOs) and governmental organisations focus on trying to address these.

At the turn of this millennium, 189 UN member states signed up to eight Millennium Development Goals to be achieved by 2015 (*see* Figure 9.2).

The Crisp Report, 'Global Health Partnerships: The UK contribution to health in developing countries', was published in 2007 (Crisp, 2007). It recognised the need to increase the international contribution of UK professionals and institutions. The government's subsequent response outlined steps that would be taken to achieve this (DH, 2008). This included the establishment of the International Health Links Centre and International Health Links Funding Scheme to support those interested in overseas work. It also resulted in the creation of the 'Framework for NHS Involvement in International Development' (DH, 2010a). This publication outlines the various other UK policy documents on global health development, including the preceding, 'International humanitarian and health work toolkit to

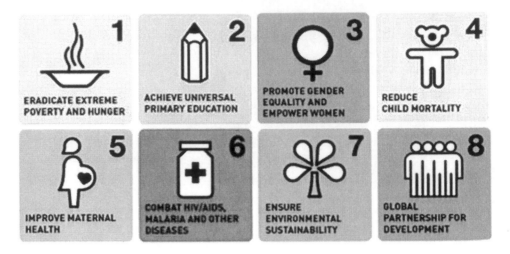

Figure 9.2: United Nations Millennium Development Goals (UN, 2000)

support good practice' (DH, 2005). Therefore alongside publications such as the BMA's 'Improving health for the world's poor – what can health professionals do?' (BMA, 2007a), these documents have been vital in raising awareness in the UK of the need to have a unified approach to improve global health. Although some of the earlier publications have been criticised for not offering practical solutions (Mabey, 2007; Whitty, Doull and Nadjm, 2007), and it can be argued that there still are significant challenges overall, these documents have taken a step towards overcoming the barriers faced by medical professionals who want to actively contribute to the improvement of worldwide health.

Skills and qualifications
Both for relief and development work you may be expected to fulfil multiple roles, as you may be one of only a few health professionals available. Hence, many NGOs will require you to have had Accident and Emergency, Paediatric, as well as Obstetrics and Gynaecology experience. NGOs will usually ask for a minimum of a three- to twelve-month commitment. It is unlikely that you will benefit from the preparation, or either party will gain enough from a period of time shorter than this. Furthermore, you will be expected to have had at least two, if not more, years of clinical experience. As an experienced doctor, you are more likely to be able to offer the necessary skills to contribute to sustainable projects.

There is a significant range of Postgraduate Certificates, Diplomas, Masters and PhDs available on subjects relevant to health professionals interested in working in a developing country. Depending on your destination, many organisations will recommend having the Diploma in Tropical Medicine & Hygiene. Among other institutions, the Liverpool School of Tropical Medicine and the London School of Hygiene and Tropical Medicine both offer this qualification, plus a diverse gamut of further relevant learning opportunities. The process of gaining such a qualification will often be an international experience in itself, due not only to the subjects covered, but also to the fact that these courses attract many overseas graduates from an assortment of professional backgrounds including doctors, nurses, health managers, researchers and non-governmental organisation staff. This inevitably enhances the opportunity to learn from each other's skills, experience and perspectives.

If invited to do so, teaching has the advantage that it can facilitate the development of local health professionals. In view of this, if you have not already done so, it may be helpful to consider investing in a postgraduate qualification in medical education (*see* Chapter 8: Teaching in general practice).

You may also consider completing a Diploma in Travel Medicine. This is intended to serve you in your work in the UK however, it is also likely to be beneficial overseas. Among numerous others, further relevant options to consider may include an MSc in Public Health, Global Health, International Primary Care, the Diploma in the Medical Care of Catastrophes, from the Royal Society of Apothecaries or perhaps qualifications in epidemiology, malnutrition, development or humanitarian emergencies. The following websites may be helpful to find the qualification or institution you need: www.prospects.ac.uk (UK), www.troped.org (International). RedR is also an example of an international charity that runs training programmes in humanitarian care (www.redr.org.uk).

Refugees and asylum seekers

If you are interested in healthcare issues that affect those who for political reasons have fled their country, working with refugees and asylum seekers in the UK is a unique opportunity to learn more about individual predicaments and about human rights in general. Volunteering offers a way to help people who may be victims of oppression or torture. In the process, you will gain a better understanding of the conflicts that many countries face and gain skills to help you in your daily clinical work.

The Medical Foundation for the Care of Victims of Torture (www.torture care.org.uk) is a human rights organisation that aims to help survivors of torture. It relies on the work of volunteer doctors and other health professionals to offer initial medical assessment and individual casework, as well as individual and group counselling. Where needed, volunteer doctors also write medico-legal reports which document the physical or psychological evidence of torture. These are then used by courts as expert witness reports in asylum claims. The work can potentially make the difference between a person gaining asylum in the UK or being deported. The Refugee Council also offers opportunities to volunteer (www.refugeecouncil.org.uk). The BMA, Medact (*see* Appendix) and the Refugee Healthcare Professionals Programme (www.rose.nhs.uk) also offer support services for refugee doctors.

Research

Research networks exist both nationally and internationally. These can act as a forum to explore research ideas and present research in progress. They can also enable the development of research skills, in addition to uniting researchers to create fruitful collaborations, and raising the profile of the need for primary care research.

The types of international research linked to primary care can be enormously varied and may include areas such as the study of the delivery of primary healthcare, health economics, policy, epidemiology and anthropology. Similar to service delivery in developing countries, it is important that research is led by local communities and is ethically sound. Also, that the research is undertaken with policymakers in mind, with thought being given as to how the potential findings may be used.

Various research funding bodies, such as the Medical Research Council (www.mrc.ac.uk), the Economic and Social Research Council (www.esrc. ac.uk) and the Wellcome Trust (www.wellcome.ac.uk), offer grants for international research. The NHS National Institute for Health Research (www. nihr.ac.uk) also has funding opportunities for trainees and GPs to undertake a Masters or PhD. In addition, several individual academic institutions and universities can offer funding or signpost you to relevant funding bodies. You can find a list of academic primary care departments through the UKs Society of Academic Primary Care (www.sapc.ac.uk).

The European General Practice Research Network (EGPRN) (www.egprn. org) forms part of the WONCA Europe network. EGPRN holds biannual meetings which are based on topical research themes. The North American Primary Care Research Group (NAPCRG) (www.napcrg.org) is another example of an international primary care research network.

International health policy

In 2008, the World Health Organization (WHO) through the publication of the annual world health report entitled, 'Primary Care, Now More than Ever' (WHO, 2008) underlined the importance of reorienting the direction of healthcare provision across the world towards that of primary care. Based in Geneva, and with offices across the world, the WHO aims to guide global health issues within the United Nations. It may seem a world away from work as a GP, however you have first-hand experience of what it means to be a clinician and thus, how policies in reality may affect patient care. This gives you a unique advantage with which to bridge the gap that often exists between clinicians, researchers and policymakers. There are various qualifications in health policy available across numerous UK and international academic institutions that may help guide a career in this direction. There are also currently opportunities to undertake internships at the WHO, although applicants must be enrolled in a degree programme in a graduate school (second university degree or higher) during the internship. The London School of Economics and Political Science, and the London School of Hygiene and Tropical Medicine offer qualifications in Health Policy and are the UK base for the European Observatory on Health Systems and Policies. This European partnership promotes evidence-based health policy-making through the study of healthcare systems. International legislation and guidance from the European Union, in addition to that of the WHO, also increasingly influences UK policy.

The Department for International Development (DIFD) is responsible for managing Britain's aid budget. To do this, it works with charities, businesses and international organisations such as the UN agencies, World Bank and European Commission. Other UK governmental departments, including the Department of Health's international division and Foreign and Commonwealth Office (FCO), are also involved in guiding health-related international policy. The National Institute for Health and Clinical Excellence (NICE) already has an international branch that aims to provide guidance to overseas governments on health policies that could be implemented locally.

Outlined in the Appendix, you will find various professional bodies and NGOs that are important actors in influencing national and international health policy. Independent think tanks such as the Nuffield Trust and King's Fund also offer insight into both national and international health policy issues.

Expedition medicine

Expeditions can range in length from a few days to over one year. They can encompass high-altitude mountain medicine, deep-sea diving expeditions, intrepid Amazon jungle exploration, desert treks or adventurous Antarctic investigations. Your potential patients could be teenagers on a social development programme, scientists carrying out research, a television crew or even a team of Guinness Book of Record breakers!

Although many expeditions may not require more than treating a few blisters and some re-hydration salts, for a case of traveller's diarrhoea, if something does goes wrong, you and the kit you have are potentially all that will save someone's life, or at least keep them stable until help arrives. You may also be expected to undertake a risk assessment for the expedition, including planning how to manage an emergency situation and prepare the equipment needed. In view of this, you will probably need extra preparation beyond what your daily work entails. This may mean refreshing your A&E skills or learning about the potential medical complications of climate and physical extremes. Furthermore, you may be called upon as a team member beyond your capacity as a doctor. Therefore leadership, diplomacy, orienteering, language and even 4×4 driving skills may come in handy, although not necessarily in that order!

There are several courses which run across the UK and overseas specialising in expedition medicine. Most of these are extremely hands-on, with mock emergency situations in rural areas. Expedition Medicine (www.expeditionmedicine.co.uk) and Wilderness Medical Training (www.wildernessmedicaltraining.co.uk) run such courses. There are also a variety of publications on the subject, including an Oxford Handbook of Expedition and Wilderness Medicine. The Royal Geographical Society (www.rgs.org) publishes a regular bulletin of expedition vacancies. Charity expedition organisations such as Raleigh (www.raleighinternational.org) are often looking for doctors who are essential for the community-based development, adventure and environmental projects they run as a youth development programme. The British Travel Health Association (www.btha.org) and Faculty of Travel Medicine (www.rcpsg.ac.uk) can be useful sources of information. The Wilderness Medical Society, although based in the USA, has some UK affiliations (www.wms.org). To consolidate your learning, you can even sit the Diploma of Mountain Medicine (www.medex.org.uk).

Planes, trains and... ships

If a patient falls ill or has a significant accident while overseas (and has travel insurance) you may be required to repatriate them to their home, as the accompanying doctor. Assignments usually involve a one to six day-long round trip escorting your patient back home on a commercial flight or, occasionally, a private jet. Due to the nature of the job you must be flexible and available at the drop of a hat, and you will need to feel confident about being the responsible doctor on the plane. However, in return you will have the opportunity to collect some air miles, perhaps fly business class, see a new country and be a friendly face for a grateful patient. Healix (www.healix.com), Europe Assistance (www.europ-assistance.co.uk) and International SOS (www.internationalsos.com), are examples of a few companies that may employ you to do this.

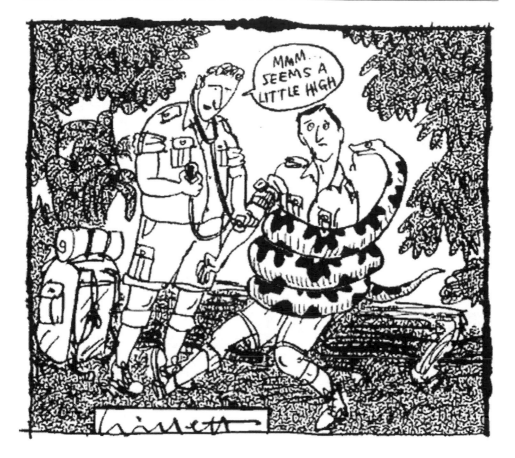

Figure 9.3: Careers – expedition medicine © Malcolm Willett & BMJ

If flying is not your thing, you may choose to work as a train's doctor. Most opportunities to do so are on board luxury private trains, some of which are steam trains. These often cater for very wealthy but ageing passengers. It is probable that you will be the only doctor on board, hence, similar to working on a plane, this may not be for the fainthearted or inexperienced. On saying this, the remoteness and beauty of routes such as the Trans-Siberian Express, Silk Road or Arctic Circle will undoubtedly make it worthwhile.

If you fancy your sea legs, cruise ships can carry around 2000–4000 passengers, some up to 5400, not dissimilar to a medium-sized practice population. However, working as ship's doctor may offer a real change of setting. In addition to routine GP work, you may be faced with unusual bites and stings, a deteriorating patient with mental illness and nail-biting decisions as to whether to make a call to ask the captain to turn the ship around. Most contracts are for at least four months. In addition to your qualifications as a GP, as with working on a plane or train, you are likely to be expected to have the various advanced life support certificates that exist.

Large ships with over 1500 passengers will usually have at least two doctors and three to four nurses, and will be fully kitted out with all you may need to treat your patients as a GP. Some even have a mini-hospital with several beds, X-ray machine, operating theatre and even intensive care unit. These can link to major hospitals in the US via satellite, creating a 'telemedicine virtual ER' whereby critical care is conducted by a specialist remotely!

If working as a ship's doctor, the chances are you will probably be expected to wear a uniform. Whether this takes your fancy or not is a matter of personal opinion, however, you will certainly earn a respectable salary

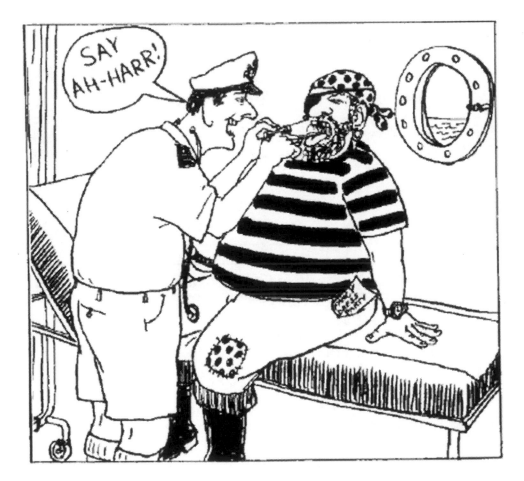

Figure 9.4: Careers: become a ship's doctor © Malcolm Willett & BMJ

to see the world and even have the opportunity to sit at the captain's table! Ocean Opportunities (www.oceanopportunities.com) and Cruise Ship Jobs (www.cruiseshipjob.com) are examples of recruitment agencies.

Fixed posts overseas

If you would like to obtain a fixed post overseas you will need to explore the processes required for your qualifications to be recognised, secure medical indemnity requirements, establish what structures exist for continuing professional development and what to do if, and when, you wish to return to the UK. If the country you plan to work in is not an English speaking country, it will be vital that you learn the local language. By doing so, you will not only be able to communicate with your patients and colleagues, but you will also gain a better understanding of the culture and society. A simple google search should give rise to medical language courses in the most commonly spoken languages worldwide.

EU regulations have made the freedom of movement for doctors in Europe much easier. The BMA International Department has produced a number of detailed papers on this subject including, 'Opportunities for doctors within the European Economic Area' (BMA, 2006) which also offers an interesting introduction to the various healthcare systems across Europe, as well as the, 'Guide to working abroad', 'GPs Working Overseas' and 'Overseas Contracts'.

You may also be able to access information from the relevant embassy or medical college. In addition, the Foreign and Commonwealth Office may provide helpful guidance. BMJ Careers (www.careers.bmj.com) regularly has listings of international posts.

The NHS; an international melting pot

The NHS itself, as the fourth largest employer in the world and the largest publicly-funded health system, is made up of professionals from across the globe that, due to a range of 'push' and 'pull' factors, have come to work in the UK (Crisp, 2010). The pros and cons of the impact of this on global health must be borne in mind, particularly the UK's contribution to the 'brain-drain'. The diversity of health professionals who have come to work in the UK has, however, undoubtedly added to the richness of the NHS. Hence, remember, you may need look no further than your colleagues to learn about medicine outside the UK and that diaspora groups in the UK can often be the key to establishing successful global partnerships.

Finally...

Write about your experience! Whether you twitter, blog, use an e-portfolio or keep an old fashioned diary, the reasons for doing this are threefold. Firstly, by keeping a meticulous record of the activities you have undertaken, you will build a professional portfolio of work, which alongside thoughtful reflection will help you learn in addition to helping with revalidation and future job interviews. Secondly, publishing your experience through the internet, in medical journals, or even presenting it back home in your surgery will allow others to see what you have witnessed and discover what you have learned. Thirdly, keep a record of it for yourself as you will look back on your experience with fondness, and perhaps be tempted to do it again!

Despite all the differences you may have encountered wherever you have been in the world, when you sit with a patient in a consultation, the objective and emotions felt are undoubtedly similar.

Organisations with International Primary Care Links

RCGP

www.rcgp.org.uk

The Royal College of General Practitioners' International Department manages the RCGP International Development programme and the MRCGP International Examination. It provides services to overseas members and provides RCGP representation at international meetings. It also facilitates dialogue and exchange through study visits to the UK and international travel scholarships. The recently formed Junior International Committee focuses on facilitating Associates in Training and First 5 GPs (within 5 years of completion of training) participation in international activities.

WONCA World

www.globalfamilydoctor.com

The World Organisation of National Colleges, Academies and Academic Associations of General Practitioners, otherwise known as the World Organisation of Family Doctors or WONCA for short, was established in 1972. As the name implies, WONCA is made up of national colleges of General Practitioners, currently from over 100 countries. It is primarily concerned with education, research and standards of practice. WONCA world hosts a triennial worldwide conference. It also hosts working parties on quality, rural family medicine, health behaviour, mental health, environment, elderly care and women in family medicine among others. WONCA world has councils in seven regions across the world, including WONCA Europe. The RCGP represents UK GPs in WONCA.

WONCA Europe

www.woncaeurope.org

WONCA Europe holds an annual conference which usually takes place over three days and plays host to a myriad of workshops, lectures and poster presentations. WONCA Europe also publishes the *European Journal of General Practice*. The European Academy of Teachers in General Practice (EURACT) (www.euract.org), European General Practice Research Network (EGPRN) (www.egprn.org), European Association for Quality in General Practice (EQuiP) (www.equip.ch), European Network for Prevention and Health Promotion (www.europrev.org) and European Rural and Isolated General Practitioners Association (EURIPA) (www.euripa.org) all form part of the wider WONCA Europe network. In conjunction with EURACT, WONCA Europe created the European Definition of Family Medicine and core competencies on which the RCGP curriculum is based (Figure 9.5). WONCA Europe also links the following special interest groups: International Primary Care Respiratory Group (IPCRG) (www.theipcrg.org), European Primary Care Cardiovascular Society (EPCCS) (www.epccs.eu), European Society for Primary Care Gastroenterology (ESPCG) (www.espcg.eu), Primary Care Diabetes Europe (PCDE) (www.pcdeurope.org)

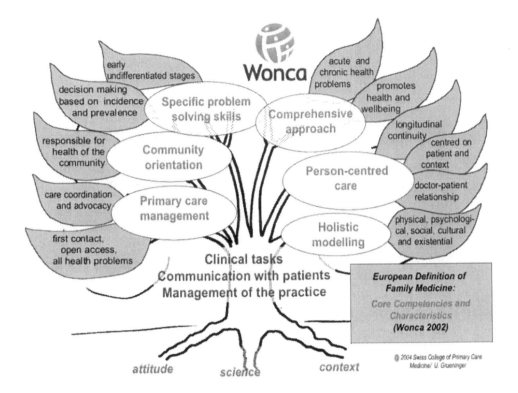

Figure 9.5: The European Definition of Family Medicine (WONCA, 2002), with permission © Swiss College of Primary Care Medicine, 2004

The Vasco da Gama Movement (VdGM)

www.vdgm.eu

VdGM is WONCA Europe's working group for young and future General Practitioners. It is open to GP trainees and GPs within five years of completion of training. In collaboration with EURACT, VdGM runs the *'Hippokrates Exchange Programme'*. This consists of hosting or visiting a foreign GP for a one- to two-week-long observational placement. The exchange offers a unique, first-hand opportunity to learn about another primary healthcare system, and can be a steppingstone to further international experiences. VdGM also offers an introduction to research and education and training opportunities in international primary care.

International Forum of the Academy of Medical Royal Colleges (AoMRC)

www.aomrc.org.uk

The International Forum of the AoMRC was set up in 1998 to bring together those involved in international activity from medical, nursing, industrial and non-governmental organisations (NGOs). The Forum aims to co-ordinate the international activities of the Royal Colleges to help improve global health, through education and training.

Alma Mata

www.almamata.net

Alma Mata is a UK-based Global Health Network. Its objective is to facilitate the development of clearer pathways for postgraduate education and careers in international health. It aims to do this through publications, lectures, conferences and by acting as a forum for the sharing of research and ideas.

IFMSA and Medsin

www.ifmsa.org www.medsin.org

The International Federation of Medical Students' Associations (IFMSA), founded in 1951, is recognised within the UN and the WHO as the International Forum for medical students. It exists to serve medical students all over the world and is represented by 'Medsin' in the UK. Among various projects, the IFMSA hosts worldwide international clinical and research exchanges.

Medact

www.medact.org

Medact is a UK-based global charity made up of health professionals. By campaigning and lobbying, it undertakes education, research and advocacy roles related to health issues resulting from conflict, development and environmental changes.

Royal Society of Medicine

www.rsm.ac.uk

Established 200 years ago, the Royal Society of Medicine (RSM) is an independent organisation. It provides continuing medical education (CME) for numerous specialties. The RSM's Catastrophe and Conflict Forum is aimed at humanitarian aid workers of all skills and specialities. The RSM now also offers increasing Global Health related events and provide a specific website for those interested in contributing to the Global Health agenda.

The European Forum for Primary Care

www.euprimarycare.org

Formed in 2005, the European Forum for Primary Care aims to improve health through promoting strong primary care. It aims to link clinicians, health policy makers, and researchers from local to international level, to provide evidence to guide primary care focused policy.

The Association for Medical Education in Europe (AMEE)

www.amee.org

Founded in 1972 in Copenhagen, AMEE's aim is to nurture dialogue between medical educators and to help promote national associations for medical education in Europe. AMEE is the European regional association of the World Federation for Medical Education.

European Union of General Practitioners (UEMO)

www.uemo.org

UEMO was established in 1967. It is a political organisation that represents GPs' interests in the EU. UEMO is the European equivalent of the General Practitioners' Committee of the BMA and is primarily concerned with the terms and conditions under which GPs work.

Permanent Working Group of European Junior Doctors (PWG)

www.juniordoctors.eu

The PWG's principal objectives include the protection of the interests of junior doctors in Europe, improvement of relations between its member organisations and the narrowing of the gap between junior doctors of the European Union and those of other European countries. It has been in existence since 1976.

The Standing Committee of European Doctors or *Comité Permanent des Médecins Européens* (CPME)

www.cpme.be

The CPME, composed of the National Medical Associations of the European Union (EU), aims to promote freedom of movement for doctors within the EU, as well as a high standard of medical training, practice and healthcare.

Examples of Non-Governmental Organisations involved in international development and/or relief work

➤ International Service   www.internationalservice.org.uk

➤ Médecins du Monde or Doctors of the World   www.doctorsoftheworld.org.uk

➤ Médecins Sans Frontières (MSF)   www.msf.org.uk

➤ Merlin   www.merlin.org.uk

➤ Progressio   www.progressio.org.uk

➤ RedR UK   www.redr.org.uk

➤ Skillshare International   www.skillshare.org

➤ Student Partnership Worldwide   www.spw.org

➤ Voluntary Service Overseas (VSO)   www.vso.org.uk

As well as countless NGOs offering development or relief work, the United Nations offers a volunteer programme (www.unv.org). The International Red Cross also offer opportunities for healthcare professionals to work for them (www.icrc.org).

For a detailed list of international institutional partnerships, NGOs, funding opportunities and guidance on international development work, the International Health Links Centre (www.ihlc.org.uk) and International Health Links Funding Scheme hosted by the Tropical Health & Education Trust (www.thet.org) as well as the British Council all offer comprehensive guidance.

Acknowledgements

Many thanks to Nick Banatvala, Simon Brownleader, Nadja van Ginneken, Ueli Grueninger, Patrick Kiernan, Steve Mowle, Mike Pringle, Abi Smith and Annette Steele.

References

Banatvala N, Macklow-Smith A. Integrating overseas work with an NHS career. *BMJ.* 1997a; **314**(7093).

Banatvala N, Macklow-Smith A. Bringing it back to Blighty. *BMJ.* 1997b; **314**(7094).

BMA. *Opportunities for Doctors within the European Economic Area.* 2006. [Online]. Available at: www.bma.org.uk/international/working_abroad/EEA.jsp (accessed 21 May 2011).

BMA. *Improving health for the world's poor: what can health professionals do?* 2007a. [Online]. Available at: www.bma.org.uk/ni/international/globalhealth/ Improvinghealth.jsp (accessed 21 May 2011).

BMA. *Broadening your horizons: a guide to taking time out to work and train in developing countries.* 2009a. [Online]. Available at: www.bma.org.uk/inter national/working_abroad/broadeningyourhorizons.jsp (accessed 21 May 2011).

BMA. *Ethics and medical electives in resource-poor countries: A toolkit.* 2009b. [Online]. Available at: www.bma.org.uk/careers/medical_education/medi calelectivestoolkit.jsp (accessed 21 May 2010).

Crawford L. MMC and overseas work. *BMJ Careers.* 2009; **338**(7688).

Crisp N. *Global Health Partnerships: The UK contribution to health in developing countries.* 2007. [Online]. Available at: www.dh.gov.uk/en/Publication sandstatistics/Publications/PublicationsPolicyAndGuidance/DH_065374 (accessed 21 May 2011).

Crisp N. *Turning the World Upside Down.* London: The RSM Press Ltd; 2010.

Davis D. Education and debate: Continuing medical education: Global health, global learning. *BMJ.* 1998; **316**(7128): 385–9.

DH. *International humanitarian and health work: toolkit to support good practice.* 2005. [Online]. Available at: www.dh.gov.uk/en/Publicationsandstatistics/ Publications/PublicationsPolicyAndGuidance/Browsable/DH_4102935 (accessed 21 May 2011).

DH. *Global health partnerships: the UK contribution to health in developing countries – the Government response.* 2008. [Online]. Available at: www.dh.gov.uk/ en/Publicationsandstatistics/Publications/PublicationsPolicyAndGuidance/ DH_083509 (accessed 21 May 2011).

DH. *International health: Department of Health objectives and ways of working.* 2009. [Online]. Available at: www.dh.gov.uk/prod_consum_dh/groups/ dh_digitalassets/documents/digitalasset/dh_106247.pdf (accessed 21 May 2011).

DH. *The Framework for NHS Involvement in International Development.* 2010a. [Online]. Available at: www.ihlc.org.uk/news/documents/framework.pdf (accessed 21 May 2011).

DH. *The Gold Guide: A Reference Guide for Postgraduate Specialty Training in the UK* (4th edn). London: Department of Health; 2010.

Grol R, Wensing M. Measuring performance quality in general practice: is international harmonization desirable? *Br J Gen Pract.* 2007; **57**(542): 691–692.

Holden J, Evans P. Is international travel useful for general practitioners? A survey of international travel scholarships. *Br J Gen Pract.* 1998; **48**(428): 1073–1075.

Horder J. The RCGP and other countries: a beginning. *Br J Gen Pract.* 1990; **40**(334): 206–209.

Johnstone P, McConnan I. Editorials: Primary health care led NHS: Learning from developing countries. *BMJ*. 1995; **311**(7010): 891–892.

Koehn P. Globalisation, migration health, and educational preparation for transnational medical encounters. *Globalization and Health*. 2006; **2**(2).

Legido-Quigley HM, Walshe K, Suñol R, *et al*. Analysis: How can quality of health care be safeguarded across the European Union? *BMJ*. 2008; **336**(7650): 920–923.

Mabey D. Editorial; Improving health for the world's poor. *BMJ*. 2007; **334**(7604): 1126.

Machin J. *The Impact of Returned International Volunteers on the UK: a scoping review*. London: Institute for Volunteering Research & VSO; 2008.

Pollit V, Martin S, Rowson M. *A Guide to Global Health Electives*. 2009. [Online]. Available at: www.ucl.ac.uk/cihd/undergraduate/elective_info/elective_pack (accessed 21 May 2011).

Spry E. Time out. *BMJ Careers*. 2008; **337**. http://careers.bmj.com/careers/advice/view-article.html?id=3075 (accessed 21 May 2011).

Tan L, Eccersley L. Teaching medicine in a developing country. *BMJ Careers*. 2005; **331**(7518).

Tooke J. *Aspiring to Excellence; Findings and Final Recommendations of the Independent Inquiry into Modernising Medical Careers*. 2008. [Online]. Available at: www.mmcinquiry.org.uk (accessed 21 May 2001).

UN. *Millennium Development Goals*. 2000. [Online]. Available at: www.un.org/millenniumgoals (accessed 21 May 2011).

Whitty CJM, Doull L, Nadjm B. Global health partnerships. *BMJ*. 2007; **334**(7594): 595–596.

WHO. *Working together for health; The world health report*. 2006. [Online]. Available at: www.who.int/whr/2006/en/ (accessed 21 May 2011).

WHO. *World Health Report: Primary Care, Now More Than Ever*. 2008. [Online]. Available at: www.who.int/whr/2008/whr08_en.pdf (accessed 21 May 2011).

WHO. *Global Health Observatory*. 2010. [Online]. Available at: apps.who.int/ghodata (accessed 21 May 2010).

WONCA. *The European Definition of Family Medicine*; 2002. [Online]. Available at: www.kollegium.ch/foto/f.las (accessed 21 May 2011).

Career profile:

Zorayda E Leopando

When did you qualify?
➤ Doctor of Medicine 1975
➤ Family Medicine Residency 1979
➤ Master in Public Health 1983 Faculty of Public Health, Mahidol University Bangkok Thailand
➤ Fellowship in Academic Family Practice 1989 Ohio State University, USA

What is your job?
I am Professor of Family and Community Medicine, College of Medicine and Philippine General Hospital, Department of Family and Community Medicine (DFCM) and Vice Chancellor for Planning and Development, at the University of the Philippines Manila.

Why and how did you choose General Practice?
I was planning to go back to the province to establish my practice and Family Medicine was the most relevant. However, I was invited to join the academic department immediately after graduating from residency training.

What do you do?
Initially, as Coordinator of the Community Health Program, I directly supervised medical interns rotating who were conducting clinics, and training mothers and volunteer health workers. I later became residency training coordinator and that was the first time we made a tracking and evaluation of the graduates and evaluated the programme.

I am also active in the Philippine Academy of Family Physicians and rose from the ranks (Director to President from 1994–1997). I was also Founding President of the Philippine Society of Teachers of Family Medicine (1986–1990, PSTFM now Foundation for Family Medicine Educators). My most significant contributions to Family Medicine in the Philippines are: setting up a Workshop on the Competencies of gatekeepers; first Strategic Planning Workshop with corresponding monitoring. I helped establish academic links for higher learning – The PSTFM-RCGP Link on enhancing primary care (1995 to 1999) and the DFCM – Department of Population Science and Primary Care of the University College London and Royal Free Medical School which focused on quality assurance, education and health financing (1999–2005). Around 25 faculty members, not only from FCM, but around the Philippines were able to observe how general practice and training and other activities are done in the UK.

Presently, there are 40 residency training programmes accredited in the Philippine Academy of Family Physicians. All medical schools have Integrated Corte Curriculum for Family and Community Medicine as a guide. The family physicians are practicing mostly in ambulatory settings, but they also have admitting privileges in hospitals.

What is the most rewarding aspect of your job?

I find it most rewarding when students appreciate the holistic approach to care provided in Family and Community Medicine and when the students and residents apply patient-centeredness, family-based and community-oriented care to patients. I have witnessed how family medicine has grown academically and in stature. Being part of the advocates to push for quality education and practice in family medicine is rewarding. The advocacy work extended up towards the Asia Pacific region and South Asia.

The Masters of Science in Clinical Medicine-Family and Community Medicine which attracted students from Indonesia and Vietnam and Saudi Arabia has been rewarding. I am co-editor in chief of *Asia Pacific Family Medicine*, the official scientific journal of Wonca Asia Pacific.

It has been humbling to be recognised internationally for what I have contributed to Family Medicine. This has included an honorary fellowship from the RCGP, Royal Australian College of General Practitioners and College of General Practitioners of Sri Lanka. I was made a Fellow of WONCA, one of three women as of now – the first one being Dr Lotte Newman from the UK and the third being Professor Cheryl Levitt of Canada.

What is the most challenging or frustrating thing about your job?

Time is not enough to do the many things we are doing. Funds are also not sufficient for all projects. It is really important to prioritise and to recruit people who will do advocacy work. Finishing the Family Medicine Textbook is one project that has been delayed. This is the textbook which will be published by the Philippine Academy of Family Physicians. The textbook shall highlight how family physicians in the Philippines are carrying out the five star role of being a healthcare provider, counsellor, educator, researcher, leader and social mobiliser. There will be three volumes, the first being on principles and philosophy and four roles. The second is on being a healthcare provider which focuses on commonly encountered problems and conditions in family medicine practice. We have subdivided this into acute and urgent, ambulatory, chronic and continuing, terminal and palliative. The third volume is on self-assessment.

If you could change one thing about your career what would it be?

I wish I could have continued to work in my practice even on a part time basis. I spent much of my time from the 1980s in advocacy for better standards in training and practice of family medicine, expanding the role of family medicine in healthcare. It is a long process.

What do you wish you knew then that you know now?

The birthing pains of Family Medicine have been experienced in almost all countries.

Reflective piece: 'Médecins Sans Frontières'

Karen Bevanmogg

12 April 2005. Aromo camp, northern Uganda. The MSF (Médecins Sans Frontières) clinic was in full swing, as it was every day except Sunday, providing basic healthcare for the camp's thirty thousand residents, displaced from their villages by the Lord's Resistance Army, who had terrorised the region for fourteen years. The government's own staff were afraid to live in the camp for fear of ambush, so we were filling in until they returned.

Patients queued patiently to be registered in the shade of the mango tree; the small concrete building was on loan from the village elders, an agreement negotiated by my predecessor. On the veranda, Stephen methodically worked his way through a line of febrile children, pricking their fingers to test for malaria; Mary dressed chronic ulcers and trauma wounds; Nelson tried to do a stocktake of pharmacy supplies; the outreach team were collecting this month's mortality figures and I was guiding our new midwife through consultation technique...

There was excitement outside and a distraught man came through, half dragging, half carrying a boy. The boy was delirious and barely conscious. Agnes, the midwife, translated his story: Peter was thirteen years old. The older man was his uncle. He had been possessed by demons for the last two days, but was well before then. Traditional medicine was not helping. Four of Peter's six siblings had died like this and the old man was terrified he would die too. It had taken a day to reach the clinic, via bus and truck.

A blood film confirmed *Falciparum malaria*, which Peter probably had in its dangerous cerebral form. David checked his observations, did a rapid examination and set up a drip. I wrote up drug and rehydration charts and gave an artemether injection. In Luo, the local tongue, Agnes explained to the uncle what was happening and why.

We returned to our respective tasks, leaving Mary to monitor Peter and call for help if he deteriorated.

Later, we moved Peter to our compound, a handful of mud tukuls (huts) where we slept during the week before returning to town at weekends. The drips continued, injections were given, observations were checked, his temperature spiked and dropped. His uncle sat with him and prayed. Peter stayed for two days. His strength returned, the demons left, he recognised his uncle and was able to complete treatment with tablets. His chances of survival had been poor, but by applying the basic principles of good medicine, I believe we pushed the odds in the right direction and probably saved his life.

General practice anywhere is about sticking to basic principles to provide good primary care: effective communication between staff, teamwork, good communication with the patients and their families, and trying to understand the context of the patient's problem. Resources, however scarce or ample, must be organised so that supplies are available when required. Staff education is essential, so that everyone knows and understands their role, not to mention sound clinical knowledge... and, in some settings, if you're the only doctor in the clinic, YOU may be responsible for it all!

As UK general practice grows increasingly protocol-driven and administration occupies more time than ever, I value how my work in Uganda (and later Zambia) presented the opportunity to confront challenges and assume responsibilities I'm unlikely to have here (despite our common principles). Forget the romantic image of Doctor in Africa. It's often a hard slog, far from home, with many frustrations along the way. I often felt out of my depth but did the best I could with what I had. Children die daily. I saw suffering that shouldn't exist. I felt angry, sad, happy, helpless!

BUT I taught colleagues skills I take for granted, learnt about logistics, organised vaccination campaigns, managed diseases I had rarely seen in England, hired and fired staff, discussed birthing methods with traditional attendants, negotiated with the local Military Commander about camp safety, pushed my boundaries and made friends for life.

However revalidation defines our continuing professional development, I would strongly recommend time abroad, in any context, to any GP who wishes to leave their comfort zone and *see* medicine and life from a different angle for a while.

Index